ADVANCES IN PATHOBIOLOGY AND MANAGEMENT OF PAGET'S DISEASE OF BONE

ADVANCES IN PATHOBIOLOGY AND MANAGEMENT OF PAGET'S DISEASE OF BONE

Edited by

SAKAMURI V. REDDY

Darby Children's Research Institute,
Medical University of South Carolina, SC,
United States

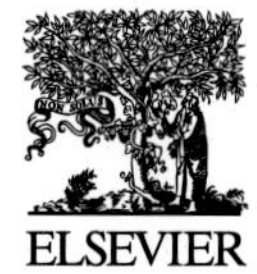

AMSTERDAM • BOSTON • HEIDELBERG • LONDON
NEW YORK • OXFORD • PARIS • SAN DIEGO
SAN FRANCISCO • SINGAPORE • SYDNEY • TOKYO
Academic Press is an imprint of Elsevier

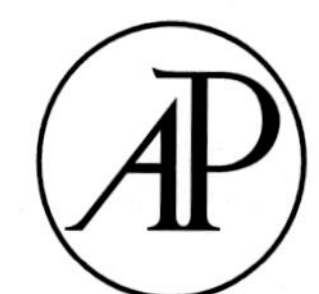

Academic Press is an imprint of Elsevier
125 London Wall, London EC2Y 5AS, UK
525 B Street, Suite 1800, San Diego, CA 92101-4495, USA
50 Hampshire Street, 5th Floor, Cambridge, MA 02139, USA
The Boulevard, Langford Lane, Kidlington, Oxford OX5 1GB, UK

British Library Cataloguing-in-Publication Data
A catalogue record for this book is available from the British Library.

Library of Congress Cataloging-in-Publication Data
A catalog record for this book is available from the Library of Congress.

ISBN: 978-0-12-805083-5

For Information on all Academic Press publications
visit our website at http://www.elsevier.com/

Publisher: Mica Haley
Acquisition Editor: Tari Broderick
Editorial Project Manager: Jeffrey Rossetti
Production Project Manager: Melissa Read
Designer: Victoria Pearson

Typeset by MPS Limited, Chennai, India

CONTENTS

LIST OF CONTRIBUTORS

Omar M.E. Albagha
Centre for Genomic and Experimental Medicine, Institute of Genetics and Molecular Medicine, University of Edinburgh, Western General Hospital, Edinburgh, United Kingdom

Jacques P. Brown
Division of Rheumatology, Department of Medicine, CHU de Québec-Université Laval, Quebec City, QC, Canada

Julie C. Crockett
Musculoskeletal Research Programme, University of Aberdeen, Aberdeen, United Kingdom

Tim Cundy
Department of Medicine, Faculty of Medical & Health Sciences, University of Auckland, Auckland, New Zealand

Deborah L. Galson
Department of Medicine, Division of Hematology-Oncology, University of Pittsburgh Cancer Institute, University of Pittsburgh School of Medicine, Pittsburgh, PA, United States

Marc F. Hansen
Center for Molecular Medicine, University of Connecticut Health Center, Boston, MA, United States

Miep H. Helfrich
Musculoskeletal Research Programme, University of Aberdeen, Aberdeen, United Kingdom

Rob Layfield
School of Life Sciences, University of Nottingham, Nottingham, United Kingdom

Laëtitia Michou
Division of Rheumatology, Department of Medicine, CHU de Québec-Université Laval, Quebec City, QC, Canada

Stuart H. Ralston
Centre for Genomic and Experimental Medicine, Institute of Genetics and Molecular Medicine, University of Edinburgh, Western General Hospital, Edinburgh, United Kingdom

Sarah L. Rea
Harry Perkins Institute of Medical Research, University of Western Australia, Nedlands, WA, Australia; Department of Endocrinology and Diabetes, Sir Charles Gairdner Hospital, Nedlands, WA, Australia

Sakamuri V. Reddy
Darby Children's Research Institute, Medical University of South Carolina, Charleston, SC, United States

Ian R. Reid
Faculty of Medical and Health Sciences, University of Auckland, Auckland, New Zealand; Auckland District Health Board, Auckland, New Zealand

G. David Roodman
Department of Medicine, Division of Hematology-Oncology, Indiana University, Indianapolis, IN, United States; Richard L. Roudebush VA Medical Center, Indianapolis, IN, United States

Margaret Seton
Division of Rheumatology, Brigham & Women's Hospital, Boston, MA, United States

Quanhong Sun
Department of Medicine, Division of Hematology-Oncology, University of Pittsburgh Cancer Institute, University of Pittsburgh School of Medicine, Pittsburgh, PA, United States

ABOUT THE EDITOR

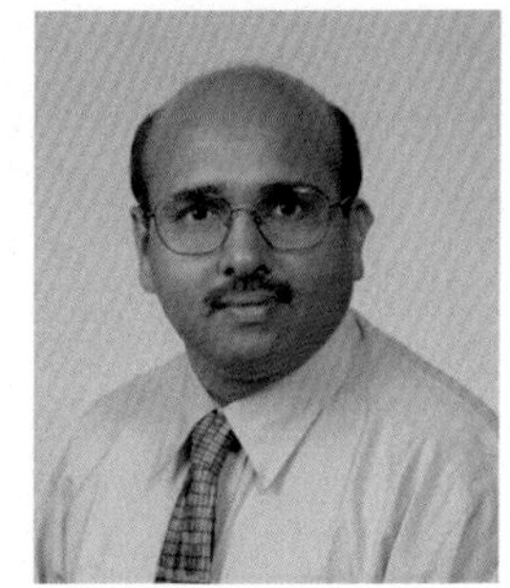

Sakamuri V. Reddy, PhD is a Professor and Director of the Osteoclast Center in the Darby Children's Research Institute at the Medical University of South Carolina (MUSC), Charleston, SC, United States. He is a member of the American Society for Bone and Mineral Research (ASBMR). Dr Reddy has over 24 years of experience in studying skeletal disorders and bone loss mechanisms. His research is focused on osteoclast biology, Paget's disease of bone, cancer metastasis to bone, and microgravity induced bone loss. He is very passionate and enthusiastic in presenting this book with recent developments in our understanding of the pathogenesis and treatment of Paget's disease of bone.

PREFACE

This book represents a comprehensive review of recent advances in our understanding of pathobiology of the Paget's disease of bone (PDB), a chronic focal skeletal disorder in older adults. The disease can occur with enlarged or deformed bones in one or more regions of the skeleton. Complications of PDB may include bone pain, osteoarthritis, femoral fractures, bowing of limbs, hearing loss, and a rare incidence of osteosarcoma. The disease has variable geographical distribution and is seen most frequently in people of Western European descent.

PDB is one of the most exaggerated examples of abnormal bone remodeling and the primary pathologic abnormality resides in the osteoclasts which resorb bone excessively, followed by osteoblast activity to form abundant poor quality new bone. Although the etiology of PDB is unclear, studies have been focused on paramyxo-viral and genetic components. A viral etiology for PDB has been suggested based on the presence of paramyxo-viral nuclear inclusions and detection of measles virus nucleocapsids (MVNP) containing several sense mutations in pagetic osteoclasts. Studies also suggest that not only the measles virus (MV), but other paramyxo-viruses such as respiratory syncytial virus or canine distemper virus, could be responsible for a slow virus infection, although others have failed to confirm these findings. In recent years, significant advancement has been made with respect to MVNP expression and pagetic osteoclast development. Also, recurrent mutations widely occur in the ubiquitin associated domain of a signaling scaffold protein, sequestosome 1 (SQSTM1/p62) in 5–10% of patients with PDB. Several other genetic loci and potential candidate genes associated with PDB are mapped; however, their contribution to PDB remains unclear. A genetic defect may favor environmental factors such as MV infection to have a potential role in pathogenesis of the disease. However, no infectious virus is isolated and the molecular basis for the persistence of the paramyxo-viral infection/expression of viral nucleocapsids in osteoclasts from patients with PDB remains unclear. The focal nature of the disease and the declining prevalence suggest that environmental factors play an important role in the pathogenesis of PDB. It is critical to determine a cause and effect relationship for the persistence of paramyxo-viral infection and genetic predisposition in patients with Paget's disease. Although PDB is generally classified as a metabolic bone disorder, it is essential to define the late onset of disease and underlying molecular mechanisms to initiate and cause progression of focal lesions. It is also important to unravel the contribution of paramyxo-viruses and genetic mutations to induce a pagetic phenotype in osteoclasts and determine what role genetics plays in marrow stroma/osteoblast function in pagetic lesions. Such studies would further clarify the etiology of PDB and advance our knowledge on skeletal biology/diseases. Bisphosphonates are now considered potent therapeutic agents for the disease; however, the future awaits new antiresorptive therapies to alleviate the risks of long-term use.

This book is dedicated in honor of Dr. Frederick R. Singer, MD, a former long-time Director of the Paget Foundation, New York, United States. He is truly a blend of science and humanity advancing this fascinating area of medical science with his noble hearted spirit.

S.V. Reddy

CHAPTER 1

Clinical Perspectives of Paget's Disease of Bone

Tim Cundy
Department of Medicine, Faculty of Medical & Health Sciences, University of Auckland, Auckland, New Zealand

INTRODUCTION

In London in November 1876 the English surgeon Sir James Paget presented to the Medical and Chirurgical Society the case of a patient that he had looked after for almost 20 years, who had an unusual deforming bone disease. He noted similar cases from the literature (the first from 1801) and suggested they were the same disorder; he published a second series of cases in 1882.

Paget was particularly struck by the enlargement of affected bones and reasoned that "only tumour, hypertrophy or chronic inflammation" could produce this effect. Thinking of parallels with chronic osteomyelitis he felt the likely pathology was "chronic inflammation" and suggested the name *osteitis deformans*. However, even by the late 19th century the eponymous name, Paget's disease, was already widely used.

We now recognize Paget's disease of bone as a focal disorder of dysregulated bone turnover that is common amongst older people, particularly those of western European descent. Although there have been significant advances in understanding the epidemiology, genetics, and molecular biology of Paget's disease, we do not yet have a complete understanding of its causes and natural history. In this chapter we examine the pathology, epidemiology, and clinical features of the disorder.

Two excellent monographs on Paget's disease are those by Ronnie Hamdy and John Kanis [1,2].

NATURAL HISTORY

There are still gaps in our knowledge of the natural history of Paget's disease. It is a lifelong disorder presenting primarily in middle-aged and older

S. V. Reddy (Ed): Advances in Pathobiology and Management of Paget's Disease of Bone.
DOI: http://dx.doi.org/10.1016/B978-0-12-805083-5.00001-4

people. It arises apparently simultaneously in one or more skeletal sites. In long bones it originates in the proximal epiphysis or metaphysis [3].

A study of 100 patients who had repeated skeletal scintiscans an average 5½ years after an initial diagnostic scan showed that none had developed new lesions [4], so the disease probably remains restricted to the bones where it originally arose. An exception to this rule is that the disease can be transferred to new skeletal sites by the use of pagetic bone for surgical bone grafting [5].

Once established, the pagetic lesion expands in size. In long bones a typical "lytic wedge," reflecting active osteoclastic resorption, can often be seen at the advancing edge—and is a sign of early disease (Fig. 1.1). In the skull this appearance is known as "osteoporosis circumscripta." The rate of progression of the disease through the skull or long bones, as estimated from serial radiographs, is in the order of 8 mm/year.

Paget's disease has characteristic radiographic appearances of varying degrees of lysis and sclerosis that reflect the histological findings of increases in both bone formation and resorption. Disease activity as assessed by plasma alkaline phosphatase (ALP) activity tends to increase slowly over time; this may reflect the expansion of lesion size, or change in disease activity. In many patients ALP activity eventually reaches a

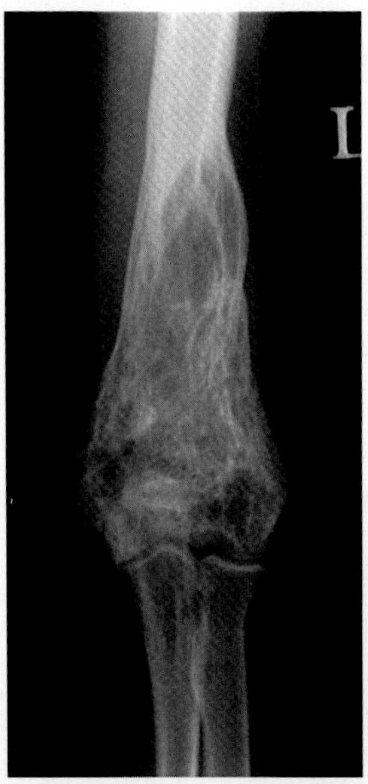

Figure 1.1 Lytic bone disease of the lower humerus.

plateau with relatively small random fluctuations. An "end-stage" disease has been described in which bone turnover declines leaving dense sclerotic bone with minimal bone turnover, but it is difficult to find convincing documentation of this happening spontaneously (see Box 1.1).

BOX 1.1

The natural history of Paget's disease is still poorly understood. It is not known how or why it starts. In long bones it spreads from the metaphyseal region through the diaphysis at about 8 mm a year. There is no evidence that it can spread from bone to bone unless pagetic tissue is used for bone grafting.

CLINICAL FEATURES AND COMPLICATIONS

In many patients Paget's disease is asymptomatic, and can remain so throughout life, but others may have symptoms for long periods before the disease is recognized (Box 1.2).

BOX 1.2

The clinical presentation can vary. A high proportion of patients have few or no symptoms. Acute complications include fracture and myelopathy. Chronic complications include bone pain, deafness (with skull involvement), and secondary osteoarthritis. In elderly patients it can be difficult to determine the contribution of Paget's disease.

Bone pain is common—typically it is worse at rest (often at night or early after rising) and is relieved by movement. Pain from osteoarthritis that is secondary to juxta-articular Paget's disease is also common. Other symptoms caused by complications include pathological fracture (which occurs most commonly in lytic disease in long bones), painful fissure fractures, bone enlargement, and deformity. Paget's disease in the skull can cause deafness (usually from involvement of the otic capsule) and increasing hat size (Figs. 1.2–1.7). Very rarely Paget's disease of the spine can cause an acute myelopathy (most commonly due to a vascular "steal"

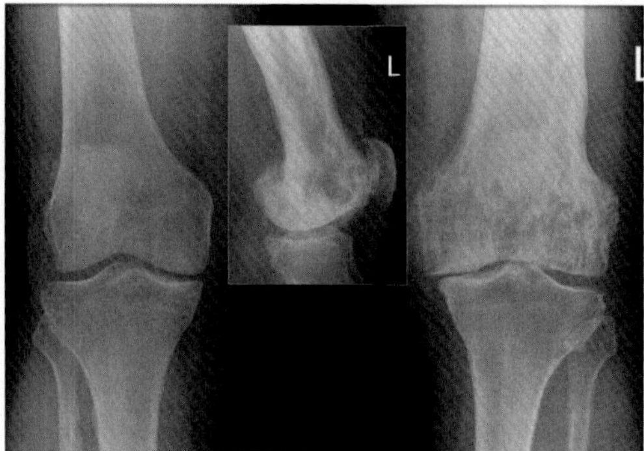

Figure 1.2 Paget's disease of the distal [L] femur. In comparison to the [R], the bone is enlarged and there is narrowing of the medial compartment of the knee joint.

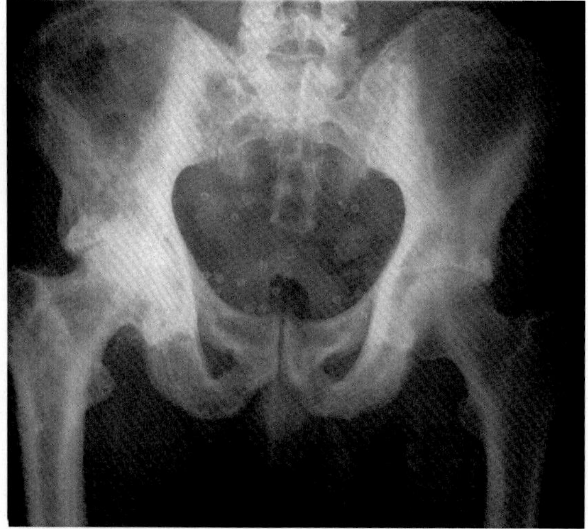

Figure 1.3 Paget's disease affecting both sides of the pelvis and the [R] femur with severe secondary osteoarthritis of the hip joint.

rather than cord compression). Any bone in the skeleton can be involved, but some more commonly than others (Table 1.1).

In a large community study [7], Paget's disease was statistically associated with back pain, osteoarthritis, hip arthroplasty, knee arthroplasty, fracture, and hearing loss.

In recent years the age at diagnosis has increased and at the same time the extent of disease has fallen. As musculoskeletal symptoms, degenerative disease of the spine, osteoarthritis, and deafness are all common in

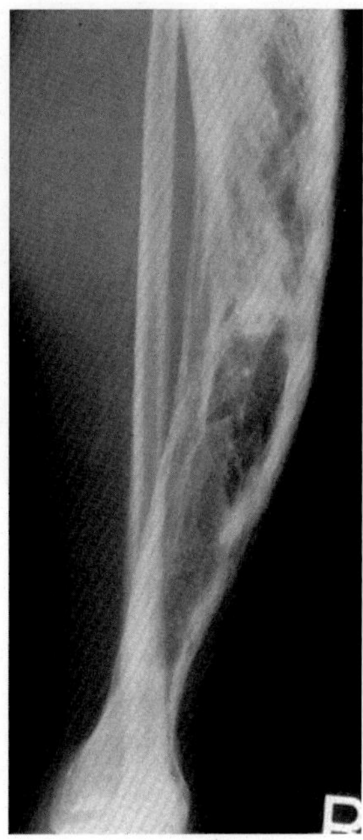

Figure 1.4 Anterior bowing deformity of the tibia.

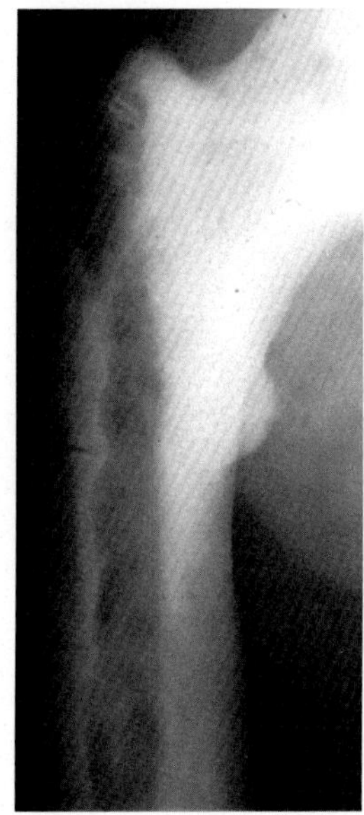

Figure 1.5 Fissure fractures on the outer femoral cortex.

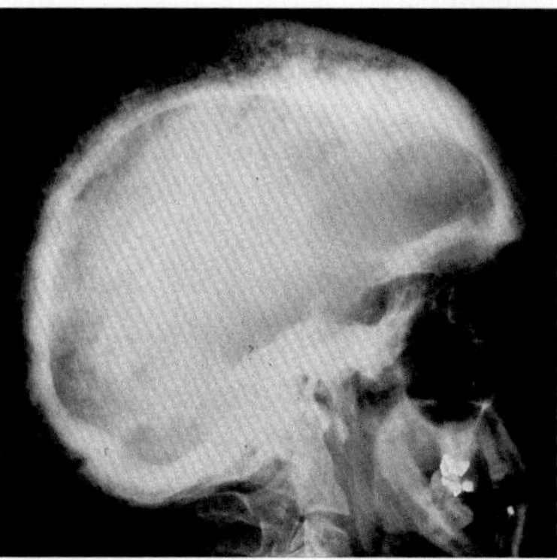

Figure 1.6 Paget's disease of the skull.

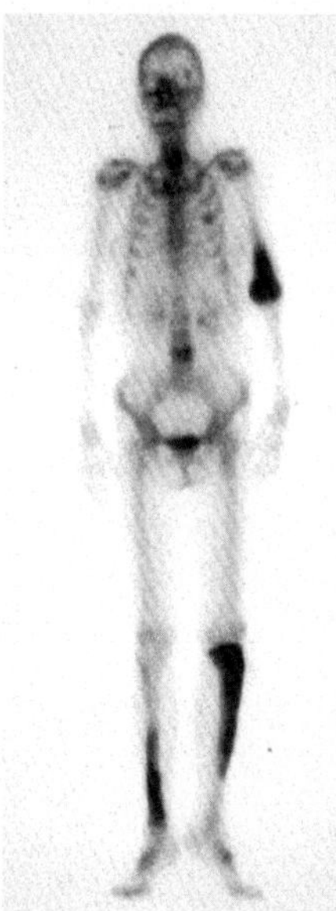

Figure 1.7 Skeletal scintiscan showing polyostotic disease affecting the distal [R] tibia, the proximal [L] tibia, proximal [L] humerus, and one lumbar vertebra.

the elderly it can be difficult in individual cases to be certain as to which symptoms are genuinely attributable to Paget's disease.

True malignancy can develop, probably the result of somatic mutation (discussed in chapter: Osteosarcoma in Paget's Disease of Bone). This feared complication typically presents as a painful enlarging mass within a pagetic bone.

Table 1.1 Bones most commonly affected by Paget's disease in decreasing order of frequency

Bone	Percentage of skeleton (per bone)[a]
Pelvis	4.5
Lumbar spine	0.65
Femur	9.5
Dorsal spine	0.3
Skull/face	17
Sacrum	2
Tibia	5
Scapula	2
Cervical vertebrae	0.2
Ribs	0.5
Sternum	0.5
Clavicle	0.5
Mandible	2
Calcaneus/foot	4
Patella	0.5
Hand bones	2
Radius	1
Fibula	1

[a]Adapted from Renier JC, Cronier P, Audran M. A new anatomic index based on current knowledge for calculating the cumulative percentage of pagetic bone. Rev Rhum (Engl Ed). 1995;52(5):355–58—this can be used to estimate the proportion of the skeleton involved on a scintiscan.

DIAGNOSIS

In symptomatic patients it may be diagnosed following pathologic fracture or investigation of musculoskeletal pain by radiography or scintigraphy. In asymptomatic patients the diagnosis is usually made incidentally either through a radiograph or scintiscan taken for some other purpose, or the finding of elevated ALP activity (with normal liver-specific enzymes) on a blood test.

The radiographic and scintigraphic appearances are characteristic (see Box 1.3 Figs. 1.2–1.7) but there can be diagnostic uncertainty in countries where Paget's disease is rare. The most important differential diagnoses are fibrous dysplasia, chronic osteomyelitis, and metastases.

In cases where the disease is picked up incidentally on radiographs it is still worth obtaining a scintiscan which will establish which other, if any, bones are involved. The disease extent can be then calculated using a measure such as the Renier index [6] (Table 1.1). This is useful particularly in research studies as an index of disease severity.

Bone biopsy is rarely required to confirm the diagnosis.

BOX 1.3 Radiographic features of Paget's disease

- Classical triad
  - Thickening of the cortex
  - Accentuation of the trabecular pattern
  - Increased size of bone
- Cyst-like areas
- Skull involvement
  - Inner and outer table involved
  - Diploic widening
    - Osteoporosis circumscripta—lysis, producing well-defined geographic lytic lesion in skull
    - "Cotton wool" appearance of thickened calvarium
    - Basilar invagination with encroachment on foramen magnum
    - Sclerosis of skull base
- Long bones
  - V-shaped defect of advancing lytic tip in diaphysis—originating from metaphysis
  - Lateral curvature of femur
  - Anterior curvature of tibia
- Pelvis
  - Thickened trabeculae in sacrum, ilium
  - Rarefaction in central portion of ilium (looks like a large lytic lesion)
  - Thickening of iliopectineal line
  - Acetabular protrusion with secondary degenerative joint disease
- Spine
  - Coarse trabeculations at periphery of bone
  - "Picture-frame vertebra"
  - Enlarged vertebral body; reinforced peripheral trabeculae/lucent center
  - "Ivory vertebra" with increased density
  - "Mickey Mouse" appearance on scintiscan

PATHOLOGY

Paget's disease is characterized by greatly accelerated remodeling activity in affected bones. The histological hallmarks include the presence of giant multinucleated osteoclasts that are actively resorbing bone. These cells contain between 3 and 30 nuclei per cell (median 9) compared to between 1 and 7 (median 3) in normal osteoclasts [2] (Fig. 1.8). Nuclear and cytoplasmic inclusion bodies can be found in electron microscopic examination of pagetic osteoclasts. The nature of these inclusions is discussed in chapters: Developmental Aspects of Pagetic Osteoclasts and Mutant SQSTM1/p62 Signaling in Paget's Disease of Bone.

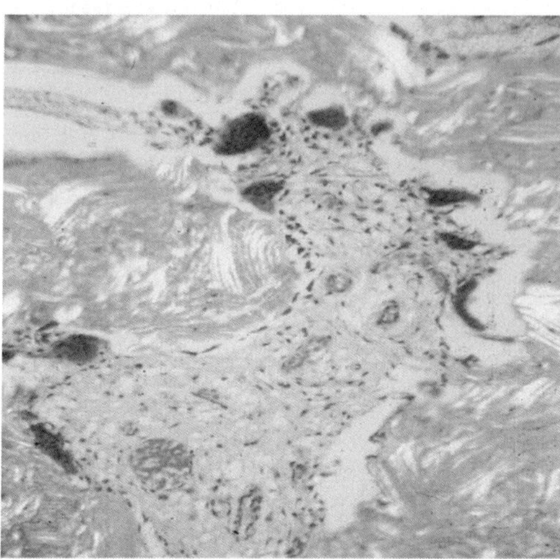

Figure 1.8 Bone histology illustrating giant multinuclear osteoclasts, marrow fibrosis, and woven bone formation.

Indices of bone formation are also high: osteoblast numbers and surface are increased, and tetracycline double-labeling indicates that tissue level bone formation rate may be increased 6–7-fold above normal levels [2,8]. Pagetic osteoblasts express a number of genes differently to nonpagetic cells [9] and osteoblast morphology also differs. The number of osteocytes (per mm^3 of bone) is also increased, and the canalicular arrangement is less organized.

The osteosclerosis seen in trabecular bone is due to increased number and thickness of trabecular elements. Increases in woven bone formation and marrow fibrosis are common but are epiphenomena of the high remodeling rate, as following successful treatment with bisphosphonates the bone formation rate also falls, and the new bone has a normal lamellar structure (see chapter: Paget's Disease of Bone: Prognosis and Complications).

BIOCHEMISTRY

The measurement of biochemical markers of bone turnover is important in both diagnosis and management. A wide variety of such markers have been used, but plasma ALP activity has the longest history, and much of our understanding of Paget's disease has been based on serial observations of ALP (Box 1.4).

BOX 1.4

Biochemical markers of bone turnover are useful in the diagnosis of Paget's disease, monitoring responses to treatment and detecting relapse. Total alkaline phosphatase is the most widely used marker, but it is often within the normal range in patients with disease of limited extent. Of the other bone markers, procollagen-1 N-propeptide performs best—values are elevated in disease of limited extent, and show the greatest changes with treatment and on relapse.

In the untreated state, ALP correlates well with the proportion of the skeleton involved, as judged by scintigraphy [2]. In healthy adults total ALP activity in plasma is derived approximately equally from liver and bone. An increased ALP is not reliable for assessing bone when other liver-derived enzymes, such as GGT, are also increased.

The newer markers of bone formation (the type I procollagen peptides P1NP and P1CP; osteocalcin and bone specific ALP) and bone resorption (breakdown products of type I collagen, and the osteoclast-derived enzymes TRAP5b and cathepsin K) do not provide additional information regarding diagnosis or effectiveness of treatment than total ALP, when the latter is clearly elevated at presentation.

However, in disease of limited extent (which is becoming increasingly the case), the extra contribution from the pagetic bone may not be sufficient to raise total ALP above the normal range. In this circumstance more specific bone markers can be helpful. P1NP seems to perform best. Pretreatment values are clearly elevated in disease of limited extent and show the greatest reduction with treatment; increases are seen early on relapse of disease [10].

EPIDEMIOLOGY

The examination of exhumed skeletons suggests that Paget's disease first appeared in Western Europe in the Roman period [11], particularly in England. The prevalence of Paget's disease in skeletons interred in a Humberside graveyard between 900 and 1850 was estimated at 2.5% [12]. From autopsies, Schmorl (1932) established that Paget's disease becomes more prevalent with increasing age, and that men are more frequently affected than women.

The prevalence is now commonly determined from surveys of radiographs (or scintiscans) in hospital settings. In the typical survey a large number of consecutive abdominal radiographs from unselected middle-aged and older subjects are reviewed for the presence of the characteristic signs of Paget's disease. This region is chosen because about 85% of subjects with Paget's disease have involvement of either lumbar spine, sacrum, pelvis, or proximal femur. Many such surveys have been carried out since the 1970s—these have demonstrated considerable between-country variation in prevalence—for example, it was more common in the United Kingdom than that in other Western European nations; and uncommon in Scandinavia, Eastern Europe, and Asia. Within European countries distinct regional variations have been reported, with the highest prevalence regions being Lancashire (England), Cabrera and Vitigudino (Spain), and Campania (Italy).

Outside Europe, the epidemiology of Paget's disease closely parallels patterns of migration from Western Europe. For example, Australia and New Zealand have a relatively high prevalence in descendants of migrants from the United Kingdom in the late 19th century, whereas it is thought to be rare amongst the indigenous peoples. Similarly, in North America, the prevalence is higher in New England than in the rest of the United States, and higher in Quebec than other Canadian provinces. Other examples of clusters apparently associated with migration include the Argentinian population of Italian descent, and the Jewish population of Recife in Brazil, of central European descent.

Not all the data supports the notion that Paget's disease is uncommon in non-European peoples. A radiographic survey in South Africa found that the prevalence in black subjects was not significantly lower than in white subjects, and as the size of the population has increased in Auckland, New Zealand we have seen more patients of Asian descent presenting with Paget's disease [13].

SECULAR CHANGE IN PAGET'S DISEASE

In a number of centers, repeat radiological prevalence surveys have been undertaken in recent years (see also Box 1.5). Compared to the estimates of 25–30 years earlier, the later studies have reported substantial falls in prevalence—about 50%—in the United Kingdom, various Western European continental centers, and New Zealand, particularly amongst younger age groups [14–16]. Criticisms of these later studies have been

BOX 1.5

Evidence for secular change in Paget's disease comes from its decreasing prevalence and reduced severity of disease in new cases (as judged by the increase in age at first presentation and reduced skeletal extent of disease). This phenomenon is also seen in offspring inheriting *SQSTM1* mutations: compared to their affected parent they have disease of later onset and attenuated severity. The prevalence of osteosarcoma, a complication of Paget's disease, is also decreasing.

that the changed use of abdominal radiographs (with greater use of diagnostic ultrasound for hepato-biliary and renal tract disorders) may have somehow selected out Paget's disease patients, and that the prevalence may have been underestimated by the inclusion of non-European subjects. However, most authorities believe this is a genuine phenomenon and a recent meta-analysis has supported this view [17].

Congruent with the idea that the prevalence is falling, is the observation that severe polyostotic disease is becoming less prevalent. Over a 30 year period in our clinic the severity of disease in newly presenting subjects (as judged by plasma ALP and disease extent on scintigraphy) fell steadily, with a reciprocal increase in the proportion of subjects having monostotic disease. Almost 40% of patients nowadays have only one bone involved [4,18]. This is not because the disease is being diagnosed earlier in life, as the mean age at diagnosis increased from 62 to 74 years over the same period. Because women have greater life expectancy than men, women now form a greater proportion of the affected population. Osteosarcoma has also become less prevalent and occurring in older patients [19].

It is uncertain when the secular change in disease severity and prevalence began, but it was noted many years ago that the proportion of death certificates mentioning Paget's disease had declined progressively in cohorts born between 1870 and 1915, as had the number of adult deaths attributed to osteosarcoma. The secular changes indicate that there is an important—as yet unidentified—environmental factor in its etiology. It is not known whether this is an organic or inorganic factor. Epidemiological studies have suggested many potential associations: with rural life and contact with animals (domestic and farm), smoking cigarettes, exposure to wood-fired heating during childhood or adolescence, and living close to a mine.

Familial Paget's disease is strongly associated with mutations in the gene *SQSTM1* and patients with such mutations typically have a more severe clinical phenotype (see chapter: Genetics of Paget's Disease of Bone). However, even amongst this group there is evidence of secular change. In a scintigraphic study of adults who had inherited *SQSTM1* mutations from affected parents, we found that the disease was emerging at least 10 years later and in a substantially attenuated form compared to their parents [20,21].

REFERENCES

[1] Hamdy RC. Paget's disease of bone: assessment and management. Connecticut: Praeger Publishers; 1981.
[2] Kanis JA. Pathophysiology and treatment of Paget's disease of bone. London: Martin Dunitz Ltd; 1991.
[3] Renier JC, Leroy E, Audran M. The initial site of bone lesions in Paget's disease—a review of two hundred cases. Rev Rhum 1996;63(11):823–9.
[4] Haddaway MJ, Davie MW, McCall IW, et al. Effect of age and gender on the number and distribution of sites in Paget's disease of bone. Br J Radiol 2007;80:523–6.
[5] Cundy T, Bolland M. Paget disease of bone. Trends Endocrinol Metab 2008;19 (7):246–53.
[6] Renier JC, Cronier P, Audran M. A new anatomic index based on current knowledge for calculating the cumulative percentage of pagetic bone. Rev Rhum (Engl Ed) 1995;52(5):355–8.
[7] Van Staa TP, Selby P, Leufkens HG, et al. Incidence and natural history of Paget's disease of bone in England and Wales. J Bone Miner Res 2002;17(3):465–71.
[8] Seitz S, Priemel M, Zustin J, et al. Paget's disease of bone: histologic analysis of 754 patients. J Bone Miner Res 2009;24(1):62–9.
[9] Naot D, Bava U, Matthews B, et al. Differential gene expression in cultured osteoblasts and bone marrow stromal cells from patients with Paget's disease of bone. J Bone Miner Res 2007;22(2):298–309.
[10] Reid IR, Davidson JS, Wattie D, et al. Comparative responses of bone turnover markers to bisphosphonate therapy in Paget's disease of bone. Bone 2004;35 (1):224–30.
[11] May S. Archeological skeletons support a northwestern European origin for Paget's disease of bone. J Bone Miner Res. 2010;25(8):1839–41.
[12] Rogers J, Jeffrey DR, Watt I. Paget's disease in an archeological population. J Bone Miner Res 2002;17(6):1127–34.
[13] Sankaran S, Naot D, Grey A, et al. Paget's disease in patients of Asian descent in New Zealand. J Bone Miner Res 2012;27(1):223–6.
[14] Cooper C, Schafheutle K, Dennison E, et al. The epidemiology of Paget's disease in Britain: is the prevalence decreasing? J Bone Miner Res 1999;14(2):192–7.
[15] Doyle T, Gunn J, Anderson G, et al. Paget's disease in New Zealand: evidence for declining prevalence. Bone 2002;31(5):616–19.
[16] Poor G, Donath J, Fornet B, Cooper C. Epidemiology of Paget's disease in Europe: the prevalence is decreasing. J Bone Miner Res 2006;21(10):1545–9.

[17] Corral-Gudino L, Borao-Cengotita-Bengoa M, Del Pino-Montes J, et al. Epidemiology of Paget's disease of bone: a systematic review and meta-analysis of secular changes. Bone 2013;55(2):347–52.
[18] Cundy HR, Gamble G, Wattie D, et al. Paget's disease of bone in New Zealand: continued decline in disease severity. Calcif Tissue Int 2004;75(5):358–64.
[19] Mangham DC, Davie MW, Grimer RJ. Sarcoma arising in Paget's disease of bone: declining incidence and increasing age at presentation. Bone 2009;44(3):431–6.
[20] Bolland MJ, Tong PC, Naot D, et al. Delayed development of Paget's disease in offspring inheriting *SQSTM1* mutations. J Bone Miner Res 2007;22(3):411–15.
[21] Cundy T, Rutland MD, Naot D, Bolland MJ. Evolution of Paget's disease of bone in adults inheriting SQSTM1 mutations. Clin Endocrinol 2015;83(3):315–19.

CHAPTER 2

Viral Etiology of Paget's Disease of Bone

Sakamuri V. Reddy
Darby Children's Research Institute, Medical University of South Carolina, Charleston, SC, United States

INTRODUCTION

Sir James Paget in 1877 first described Paget's disease of bone (PDB), or *osteitis deformans*, as chronic inflammation of bone. PDB is a focal skeletal disease that affects 2–3% of the population over the age of 55. The disease involves deformity and enlargement of single or multiple bones which include the skull, clavicles, long bones, and vertebral bodies [1]. It can be monostotic or polyostotic with bone lesions continuing to progress in size and new lesions rarely developing during the course of the disease. PDB is characterized by an increased bone resorption followed by an abundant poor quality new bone formation. The disease has variable geographic distribution with an increased incidence in people of European descent. However, the prevalence of PDB has been declining over the last several decades [2]. Patients with PDB are frequently asymptomatic, but approximately 10–15% have severe symptoms which include bone pain, fractures, secondary osteoarthritis, deafness, dental abnormalities, and neurological complications. Also, less than 1% of Paget's patients develop osteosarcoma in an affected bone. PDB is an autosomal dominant trait with genetic heterogeneity. The disease is implicated as a slow paramyxo-viral infection process, suggesting a viral etiology. However, the cause and effect relationship among genetic and viral etiologic factors in the pathophysiology of PDB remains elusive. This chapter will highlight the paramyxo-viral etiology and interactions with genetic factors associated with Paget's disease.

PARAMYXO-VIRAL ETIOLOGY

The primary abnormality in PDB resides in the bone-resorbing osteoclast cells. A viral etiology has been proposed due to an initial description of

S.V. Reddy (Ed): Advances in Pathobiology and Management of Paget's Disease of Bone.
DOI: http://dx.doi.org/10.1016/B978-0-12-805083-5.00002-6

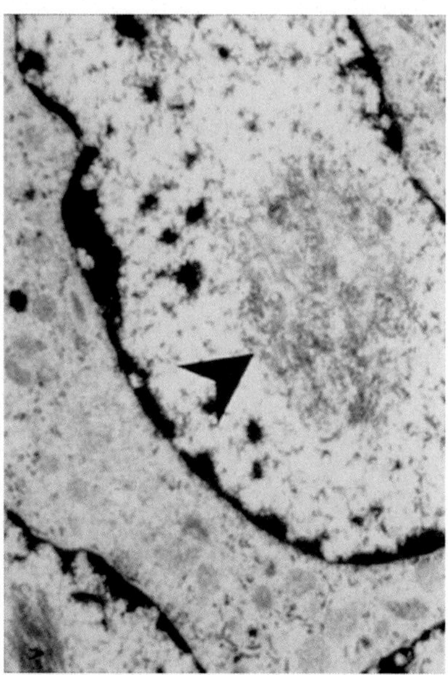

Figure 2.1 Electron microscopy analysis of paramyxo-viral nuclear inclusions in a pagetic osteoclast. The arrow points to nuclear inclusions. *Photomicrograph is courtesy of Frederick R. Singer, MD.*

nucleocapsid-like structures in the nuclei and cytoplasm of pagetic osteoclasts by electron microscopy [3]. The nuclear inclusions occur at 20–40% of osteoclasts in a pagetic bone specimen and occupy 15% of the nuclear area. The nuclear inclusions in pagetic osteoclasts closely resemble the paramyxo-viruses (Fig. 2.1). However, nuclear inclusions have not been found in osteoblasts and osteocyte cells in these patients. The paramyxo-viral-like nuclear inclusions are not unique to PDB and were reported in patients with Familial expansile osteolysis, and rarely in patients with osteopetrosis, pycnodysostosis, otosclerosis, and oxalosis. Immunohistochemical studies further identified both measles virus (MV) and respiratory syncytial virus (RSV) nucleocapsid antigens expressed in osteoclasts in Paget's patients. Similarly, mononuclear and multinucleated cells formed in pagetic bone marrow cultures demonstrated expression of paramyxo-viral nucleocapsid antigens [4]. Thus, ultrastructural cellular studies indicated PDB is associated with a slow virus infection analogous to subacute sclerosing panencephalitis due to MV infection in childhood. There is an increased incidence of Paget's disease in people with dog ownership. Canine distemper virus (CDV) nucleocapsid antigens have been detected in osteoclasts from patients with PDB [5]. Canine bone marrow cells infected with CDV developed multinucleated cells which share some of the phenotypic characteristics of pagetic osteoclasts. CDV infection to human preosteoclast cells also enhances osteoclast differentiation and bone resorption activity [6]. These cellular and molecular studies implicated paramyxo-viral etiology plays an important role in the pathogenesis of Paget's disease. Although, the presence of nuclear inclusions in pagetic osteoclasts suggested a viral etiology for Paget's disease, no infectious virus is isolated. However, the absence of budding of intact virions from the cell surface suggested that they are defective viruses [7]. Since paramyxo-viruses are RNA viruses, it is unlikely that the viral genome is integrated into the genome of the affected population. However, RSV persistence in macrophages has been shown to alter cellular gene expression profile [8]. Persistence of defective paramyxo-viruses at very low levels in focal lesions evades the immune responses in Paget's patients. Inflammation is associated with many chronic age-related diseases, such as arthritis, and may trigger an initial event to develop pagetic lesions. The familial and sporadic nature of PDB suggests that altered gene loci may predispose people to environmental factors, such as paramyxo-viruses infection and persistence to develop Paget's disease. In studies, using normal osteoclast precursors transduced with retroviral vectors expressing the measles virus nucleocapsid (MVNP) gene formed pagetic-like osteoclasts more rapidly with an increased numbers of nuclei, hypersensitivity to 1,25-dihydroxyvitamin D3 (calcitriol), and showed increased bone-resorbing capacity compared to normal osteoclasts. In contrast, MV matrix gene did not alter osteoclast phenotype [9]. Transgenic mice targeted with CD46, the human MV receptor expression to osteoclast lineage cells, demonstrated that MV infection induces pagetic phenotype in osteoclasts in vitro [10]. However, mice do not develop sustained MV infection and blocking interferon production is necessary for persistence [11]. Mice targeted with MVNP expression to the cells of the osteoclast lineage resulted in pagetic bone phenotype [12]. Conversely, human T-cell leukemia virus type 1 (HTLV-1) oncogene, *Tax* overexpression in mice resulted in high bone turnover and osteolytic bone metastasis of lymphoma tumor cells due to production of osteoclastogenic factors; however, pagetic bone phenotype was not induced [13]. These studies confer the specificity for MVNP to induce pagetic phenotype (detailed in chapter: Developmental Aspects of Pagetic Osteoclasts) in osteoclasts and suggest paramyxo-virus is an etiologic agent in the pathogenesis of

PDB [14]. However, these studies do not exclude genetic factor(s) that may play an important role in disease severity and pathogenesis.

Paramyxo-viruses are negative-sense single-stranded RNA viruses and the gene sequences within the viral genome are much conserved across the family. In situ hybridization techniques identified the presence of RNA encoding the MVNP in more than 90% of osteoclasts and other mononuclear cells in pagetic bone specimens [15]. Bone marrow cells from patients with Paget's disease showed expression of MVNP transcripts with sense mutations, which resulted in amino acid substitutions clustered at the c-terminal end. The mutations occur at a 1% rate in the total MVNP gene. Osteoclast progenitors (CFU-GM), committed preosteoclast cells, and osteoclasts from PDB patients express MVNP transcripts indicating MV infection in early osteoclast lineage cells (Fig. 2.2). MVNP transcripts were also detected in peripheral blood monocytes from Paget's patients [16]. Merchant et al., have reported MVNP expression in pagetic bone as well as pagetic osteosarcoma samples [17]. In addition to osteoclast lineage cells, MVNP expression is also detected in other hematopoietic lineage cells, such as the erythroid precursors and multipotent myeloid precursors, from these patients. Therefore, pluripotent hematopoietic stem cells which can persist for long periods of time in a quiescent phase may be the initial target and explains the chronicity of the infection [18]. Genetic predisposition may also play a role in persistence of paramyxo-viral infection in these patients. The presence of paramyxo-viral transcripts in

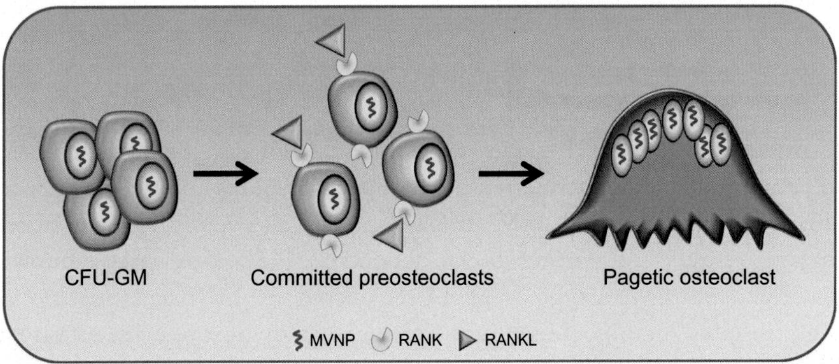

Figure 2.2 Expression of measles virus nucleocapsid (MVNP) transcripts in osteoclast lineage in PDB. RANK receptor expressed on preosteoclast cells upon interaction with RANKL results in osteoclast differentiation and bone resorption. MVNP mRNA expression is detected in early osteoclast progenitors (CFU-GM), committed preosteoclasts, and osteoclasts in patients with PDB.

osteoclast precursors and activated osteoclasts suggest a pathophysiologic role for these genes in the development of the pagetic lesions associated with the disease. However, others have been unable to detect paramyxo-viral nucleocapsid transcripts in these patients [19,20]. The contribution of other environmental factors to the pathogenesis of PDB is obscure and none other than paramyxo-viruses have been shown to induce pagetic phenotype in osteoclasts both in vitro and in vivo. Although evidence strongly supports paramyxo-viral etiology, it is still unclear in the late-onset and focal nature of Paget's disease.

VIRAL AND GENETIC INTERACTIONS

Osteoclasts in Paget's disease are characterized by increased levels of IL-6, an autocrine/paracrine factor, and c-Fos expression. Studies have shown that measles virus nucleocapsid protein (MVNP) expression in osteoclast lineage cells increases IL-6 production and transcription factors, such as c-Fos and NFATc1, critical for osteoclast differentiation [21]. MVNP expression in osteoclast precursors results in hypersensitivity to calcitriol through elevated levels of vitamin D receptor coactivator, TAF12 in PDB [22]. TANK-binding kinase 1 (TBK1) which complexes with MVNP and activates NF-kB pathways could mediate MVNP induced pagetic osteoclast formation [23]. RANK ligand (RANKL), a critical osteoclastogenic factor, is upregulated in PDB. MVNP expression in bone marrow monocytes elevated the levels of CXCL5 and FGF-2, which induce RANKL expression in stromal/preosteoblast cells [24]. Microarray (~26,000 genes) analysis of MVNP regulated gene expression profiling identified that 8.4% of genes upregulate during the osteoclast differentiation. MVNP increased immunoreceptor tyrosine-based activation motif (ITAM)-bearing signaling molecules, signal regulatory protein beta 1 (SIRPβ1), and NFAT activating protein with ITAM motif 1 (NFAM1) gene expression. SIRPβ1 interacts with DAP12, an ITAM motif containing adapter protein, which plays an important role in osteoclast differentiation. Bone marrow mononuclear cells derived from patients with PDB are associated with high level expression of SIRPβ1 and NFAM1 mRNA expression suggesting that ITAM signaling cascades may have a functional significance in MVNP induced pagetic osteoclast development [25]. Gene expression analysis studies thus indicated that MVNP upregulation of several cytokines, signaling molecules, and transcription factors plays an important role in the pathophysiology of PDB (Fig. 2.3). However, the

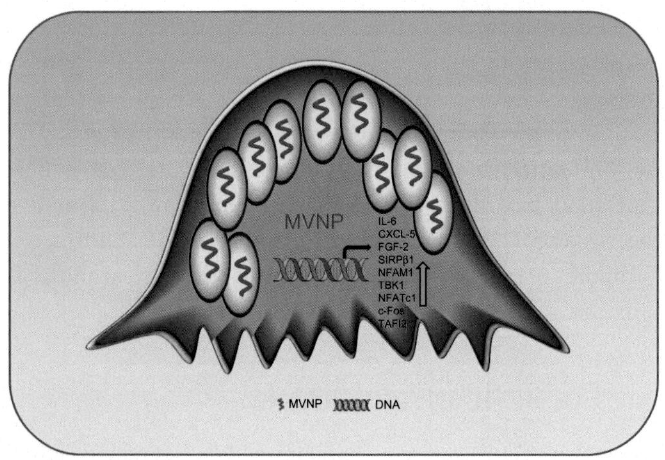

Figure 2.3 MVNP induces cytokines, signaling molecules, and transcription factors which contribute to pagetic osteoclast differentiation.

contribution of genetic factors to MVNP induced pagetic osteoclast development and pathogenesis of Paget's disease is unclear.

Sequestosome 1 (SQSTM1/p62) functions as a shuttling factor of poly-ubiquitinylated proteins for proteosomal degradation. p62 UBA domain mutation ($p62^{P392L}$) is widely identified in patients with PDB. Familial history of PDB occurs in 15–40% patients and of which only 20–30% have a p62 mutation. Thus, p62 mutations occur in 5–10% of total PDB population. Genetic linkage analysis indicated that mutations in the p62 gene do not completely account for the pathogenesis of PDB [26]. Patients with p62 mutations displayed polyostotic involvement, indicating severity of the disease. However, patients carrying a single p62 mutation showed significant intrafamilial variability in the presentation of PDB [27]. Severity of disease in family members carrying the same mutation can vary widely, and several individuals who harbor p62 mutations do not have PDB. Osteoclast precursors from patients with PDB are hypersensitive to both RANKL and calcitriol. Studies using transgenic mice which harbor the $p62^{P394L}$ mutation (equivalent to human $p62^{P392L}$) showed increased osteoclastogenic potential due to increased RANKL expression in marrow stromal cells in the bone microenvironment but do not induce Paget's disease. The osteoclast precursors from these mice are hypersensitive to RANKL but not to calcitriol [28]. p62 UBA mutant (P394L) mice develop osteopenia and upon coexpression with MVNP showed severe pagetic bone lesions [29]. Conversely, others have shown that mice with p62 (P394L) mutation have small focal lesions with increased osteoclast number, size, and some nuclear inclusions. This study also suggested that p62 mutant mice showed enhanced autophagosome formation and dysregulated autophagy, a cellular process for lysosomal degradation of damaged/dysfunctional organelles and protein aggregates [30]. Elevated levels of autophagy-related proteins were found in osteoclasts from Pagetic bone biopsies [31]. The elevated levels of autophagy in osteoclasts could be due to antiresorptive drug therapy and/or viral factors expressed in these patients. Protein aggregates are often cytotoxic and have been implicated in a wide variety of degenerative pathologic conditions, such as Alzheimer's disease. Aggregation of cellular protein(s) due to altered autophagy does not explain how the osteoclasts are long-living, hyperactive and abundant in pagetic lesions. p62 being ubiquitously expressed, the specificity of mutant p62 to cause protein aggregation in osteoclasts at focal lesions and the late onset of the disease is not addressed. In vitro studies revealed that the p62 UBA mutation (P392L) abolished interaction with the deubiquitinase, CYLD, and contributed to enhanced osteoclast development and excess bone resorption, which are associated with PDB [32]. p62 null mice have a normal skeletal phenotype with no alterations found in the trabecular size and number of osteoclasts, suggesting that basal osteoclastogenesis is not affected by p62 deficiency [33]. However, SQSTM1/p62 is neither necessary nor sufficient to cause PDB [34]. Other gene loci may be involved in the genetic predisposition and the potential role for paramyxo-virus in abnormal osteoclast development and high bone turnover associated with PDB. Mutations in the gene encoding valosin-containing protein, a multiubiquitin chain targeting factor for proteasome degradation, have been shown to cause inclusion body myopathy associated with PDB and frontotemporal dementia (IBMPFD) [35]. Genome-wide association studies in individuals without p62 mutations have further identified genetic variants such as CSF1, OPTN, and TNFRSF11A (RANK) and several other candidate genes (see chapter: Genetics of Paget's Disease of Bone) as risk factors that may predispose to Paget's disease [36,37] however, their functional role in MVNP induced pagetic osteoclast development and their contribution to the pathogenesis of PDB is yet to be elucidated (Fig. 2.4). Future studies should provide molecular insights into genetic susceptibility for paramyxoviral infection, focal lesions, and late onset of Paget's disease.

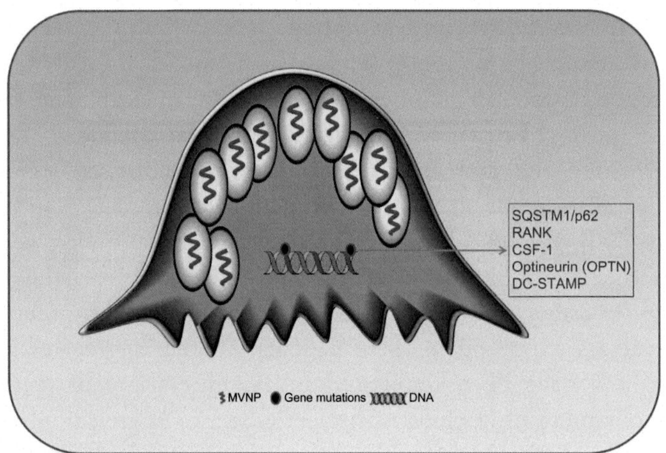

Figure 2.4 MVNP interaction with genetic factors enhances osteoclast activity in Paget's disease. Environmental factors, such as MVNP, induce pagetic osteoclast development and genetic factors, such as SQSTM1/p62 UBA mutation, contribute to enhanced osteoclast activity in PDB. Several other candidate genes (detailed in the chapter: Genetics of Paget's Disease of Bone) are potentially linked to Paget's disease; however their role in the pathophysiology of PDB remains unknown.

Acknowledgments

The author thanks Dr. Yuvaraj Sambandam for assistance with the art work.

REFERENCES

[1] Paget J. On a form of chronic inflammation of bones (Osteitis Deformans). Med Chir Trans 1877;60(37–64):39.
[2] Doyle T, Gunn J, Anderson G, Gill M, Cundy T. Paget's disease in New Zealand: evidence for declining prevalence. Bone 2002;31:616–19.
[3] Mills BG, Singer FR. Nuclear inclusions in Paget's disease of bone. Science 1976;194:201–2.
[4] Singer FR, Mills BG, Gruber HE, Windle JJ, Roodman GD. Ultrastructure of bone cels in Paget's disease of bone. J Bone Miner Res 2006;21(Suppl. 2):P51–4.
[5] Mee AP, Dixon JA, Hoyland JA, et al. Detection of canine distemper virus in 100% of Paget's disease samples by in situ-reverse transcriptase-polymerase chain reaction. Bone 1998;23:171–5.
[6] Mee AP, Sharpe PT. Dogs, distemper and Paget's disease. BioEssays 1993;15:783–9.
[7] Abe S, Ohno T, Park P, et al. Viral behavior of paracrystalline inclusions in osteoclasts of Paget's disease of bone. Ultrastruct Pathol 1995;19:455–61.
[8] Rivera-Toledo E, Gómez B. Respiratory syncytial virus persistence in macrophages alters the profile of cellular gene expression. Viruses 2012;4(12):3270–80.
[9] Kurihara N, Reddy SV, Menaa C, Anderson D, Roodman GD. Osteoclasts expressing the measles virus nucleocapsid gene display a pagetic phenotype. J Clin Invest 2000;105:607–14.

[10] Reddy SV, Kurihara N, Menaa C, et al. Osteoclasts formed by measles virus-infected osteoclast precursors from hCD46 transgenic mice express characteristics of pagetic osteoclasts. Endocrinology 2001;142:2898–905.
[11] Peng KW, Frenzke M, Myers R, et al. Biodistribution of oncolytic measles virus after intraperitoneal administration into Ifnar-CD46Ge transgenic mice. Hum Gene Ther 2003;14:1565–77.
[12] Kurihara N, Zhou H, Reddy SV, et al. Experimental models of Paget's disease. J Bone Miner Res 2006;21(Suppl. 2):P55–7.
[13] Gao L, Deng H, Zhao H, et al. HTLV-1 Tax transgenic mice developo spontaneous oseolytic bonemetastases prevented by osteoclast inhibition. Blood 2005;106:4294–302.
[14] Singer FR. Paget's disease of bone-genetic and environmental factors. Nat Rev Endocrinol 2015;11(11):662–71.
[15] Basle MF, Fournier JG, Rozenblatt S, Rebel A, Bouteille M. Measles virus RNA detected in Paget's disease bone tissue by in situ hybridization. J Gen Virol 1986;67:907–13.
[16] Reddy SV. Etiology of Paget's disease and osteoclast abnormalities. J Cell Biochem 2004;93:688–96.
[17] Merchant A, Smielewska M, Patel N, et al. Somatic mutations in SQSTM1 detected in affected tissues from patients with sporadic Paget's disease of bone. J Bone Miner Res 2009;24:484–94.
[18] Reddy SV. Etiologic factors in Paget's disease of bone. Cell Mol Life Sci 2006;63:391–8.
[19] Helfrich MH, Hobson RP, Grabowski PS, et al. A negative search for a paramyxoviral etiology of Paget's disease of bone: molecular, immunological, and ultrastructural studies in UK patients. J Bone Miner Res 2000;15:2315–29.
[20] Matthews BG, Afzal MA, Minor PD, et al. Failure to detect measles virus ribonucleic acid in bone cells from patients with Paget's disease. J Clin Endocrinol Metab 2008;93:1398–401.
[21] Shanmugarajan S, Youssef RF, Pati P, Ries WL, Rao DS, Reddy SV. Osteoclast inhibitory peptide (OIP-1) inhibits measles virus nucleocapsid protein stimulated osteoclast formation/activity. J Cell Biochem 2008;104:1500–8.
[22] Teramachi J, Hiruma Y, Ishizuka S, et al. Role of ATF7-TAF12 interactions in the vitamin D response hypersensitivity of osteoclast precursors in Paget's disease. J Bone Miner Res 2013;28:1489–500.
[23] Sun Q, Sammut B, Wang FM, et al. TBK1 mediates critical effects of measles virus nucleocapsid protein (MVNP) on pagetic osteoclast formation. J Bone Miner Res 2014;29:90–102.
[24] Sundaram K, Rao DS, Ries WL, Reddy SV. CXCL5 stimulation of RANK ligand expression in Paget's disease of bone. Lab Invest 2013;93:472–9.
[25] Sambandam Y, Sundaram K, Reddy SV. NFAM1 signaling modulates osteoclast differentition in Paget's disease of bone. ASBMR, Baltimore, MD, Oct 4–7, (Abstract #LB-M033), 2013.
[26] Helfrich MH, Hocking LJ. Genetics and aetiology of Pagetic disorders of bone. Arch Biochem Biophys 2008;473:172–82.
[27] Leach RJ, Singer FR, Ench Y, et al. Clinical and cellular phenotypes associated with sequestosome 1 (SQSTM1) mutations. J Bone Miner Res 2006;21(Suppl. 2): P45–50.
[28] Kurihara N, Hiruma Y, Zhou H, et al. Mutation of the sequestosome 1 (p62) gene increases osteoclastogenesis but does not induce Paget disease. J Clin Invest 2007;117:133–42.

[29] Kurihara N, Hiruma Y, Yamana K, et al. Contributions of the measles virus nucleocapsid gene and the SQSTM1/p62(P392L) mutation to Paget's disease. Cell Metab 2011;13:23–34.
[30] Daroszewska A, van 't Hof RJ, Rojas JA, et al. A point mutation in the ubiquitin associated domain of SQSMT1 is sufficient to cause a Paget's disease like disorder in mice. Hum Mol Genet 2011;20:2734–44.
[31] Hocking LJ, Whitehouse C, Helfrich MH. Autophagy: a new player in skeletal maintenance? J Bone Miner Res 2012;27:1439–47.
[32] Sundaram K, Shanmugarajan S, Sudhaker Rao D, Reddy SV. Mutant p62 stimulation of osteoclast differentiation in Paget's disease of bone. Endocrinology 2011;152:4180–9.
[33] Duran A, Serrano M, Leitges M, et al. The atypical PKC-interacting protein p62 is an important mediator of RANK-activated osteoclastogenesis. Dev Cell 2004;6:303–9.
[34] Seton M. Paget's disease: epidemiology and pathophysiology. Curr Osteoporos Rep 2008;6:125–9.
[35] Weihl CC, Pestronk A, Kimonis VE. Valosin-containing protein disease: inclusion body myopathy with Paget's disease of the bone and fronto-temporal dementia. Neuromuscul Disord 2009;19:308–15.
[36] Albagha OM, Visconti MR, Alonso N, et al. Genome-wide association study identifies variants at CSF1, OPTN and TNFRSF11A as genetic risk factors for Paget's disease of bone. Nat Genet 2010;42:520–4.
[37] Albagha OM. Genetics of Paget's disease of bone. BoneKEy Rep 2015;4:756.

CHAPTER 3

Genetics of Paget's Disease of Bone

Omar M.E. Albagha and Stuart H. Ralston
Centre for Genomic and Experimental Medicine, Institute of Genetics and Molecular Medicine, University of Edinburgh, Western General Hospital, Edinburgh, United Kingdom

INTRODUCTION

Paget's disease of bone (PDB) is a skeletal disorder characterized by focal areas of increased osteoclastic bone resorption coupled to increased and disorganized bone formation. Other cellular abnormalities include bone marrow fibrosis and increased vascularity of bone. Paget's disease rarely affects people below the age of 55 years but increases in incidence progressively thereafter. The most common presenting symptom is bone pain but other complications that may occur include bone deformity, pathological fracture, nerve compression syndromes and osteoarthritis. About 20% of patients who come to medical attention are asymptomatic [1]. However it is recognized that only 8–15% of patients with radiological evidence of the disease present clinically [1,2].

Paget's disease is a complex disorder. Current evidence indicates that genetic factors play a key role although it is clear that environmental triggers also modulate susceptibility and severity of the disease. In this chapter we review recent advances in understanding of the genetic factors that contribute to PDB.

IMPORTANCE OF GENETIC FACTORS

Familial clustering of PDB was first reported by in 1949 [3] but since then, many studies have provided support for the importance of heredity in the pathogenesis of PDB. Familial clustering of PDB is common and relatives of an affected person have approximately seven times greater risk of developing PDB than those in the general population [4,5]. In some families the disease follows an autosomal dominant mode of inheritance with incomplete penetrance [6–9]. Patients with PDB with no family history are

S.V. Reddy (Ed): Advances in Pathobiology and Management of Paget's Disease of Bone.
DOI: http://dx.doi.org/10.1016/B978-0-12-805083-5.00003-8

considered to have "sporadic" disease. In these cases the disease could occur as a result of isolated de novo mutations, environmental triggers, or simply due to incomplete penetrance concealing family history. It is of interest that the prevalence of PDB varies substantially between ethnic groups. Paget's is common in the UK and in other European countries such as Italy, Spain, and France and is also common in countries like Australia, New Zealand, and in Quebec, Canada where there has been migration from high prevalence countries. These observations provide further support for the importance of genetic factors in PDB.

In addition to classical PDB, many rare PDB-like syndromes have been identified including expansile skeletal hyperphosphatasia, familial expansile osteolysis and juvenile PDB. These are discussed elsewhere in this book.

Over recent years, genetic linkage studies in families coupled with genome-wide association studies (GWAS) have identified several genes and chromosomal loci which predispose to PDB; these are described in more detail below [10–13].

SQSTM1

Mutations in *SQSTM1* were identified in PDB through linkage studies in families and positional cloning. Genome-wide linkage studies in the French-Canadian and UK populations revealed evidence of susceptibility loci on chromosomes 5q31, 5q35, and 10p13 and 2q36 [8,9,14]. The strongest evidence for linkage was reported for the 5q35 locus which was confirmed by two independent studies [8,9]. Subsequent positional cloning studies showed that mutations in *SQSTM1* gene were responsible for 5q35-linked PDB. The first mutation to be described was a proline to leucine amino acid change at codon 392 (P392L) in the French-Canadian population [8] and subsequently several other mutations were identified in the UBA domain in the UK population [11]. To date more than 23 different mutations have been identified in *SQSTM1* in patients with PDB and most affect the UBA domain [15,16]. The *SQSTM1* gene encodes p62 which is an adapter protein that binds ubiquitin and plays an important role in the NFκB signaling pathway as discussed elsewhere in this book. The mechanism by which mutations in the *SQSTM1* gene lead to PDB development is still unclear, but current evidence suggests that the causal mutations impair the ability of p62 to recruit CYLD to the intracellular signaling complex downstream of the RANK receptor

[17,18] leading to enhanced NFκB signaling and increased sensitivity of osteoclasts precursors to RANKL [19].

The status of the 5q31 locus for Paget's identified in the French-Canadian population remains unclear. Although the linkage peak was significant at a genome-wide level, no causal gene has so far been identified. Linkage analysis of UK families with PDB not related to *SQSTM1* mutations confirmed the status of the 10p13 locus as an important susceptibility region for the disease, whereas association with the 2q36 locus was no longer significant indicating that it was likely a false positive signal.

TNFRSF11B

The *TNFRSF11B* gene encodes osteoprotegerin, an inhibitor of bone resorption which is a decoy receptor for RANKL [20,21]. Loss of function mutations in *TNFRSF11B* cause the rare syndrome of juvenile PDB [22,23]. Based on this observation, several investigators have investigated the hypothesis that genetic variants in the *TNFRSF11B* gene might predispose to classical PDB. In one study a nonsynonymous coding variant resulting in a lysine–asparagine substitution at codon 3 of the OPG signal peptide (K3N) was reported to be associated with an increased risk of PDB in a UK population [24]. Subsequently this association was confirmed by Beyens who intriguingly found that the association was restricted to female patients [25]. The status of OPG as a predisposing factor for PDB is unclear at present, however, since the *TNFRSF11B* locus did not emerge as a significant determinant of susceptibility in GWAS studies. Therefore, further studies will be required to confirm or refute the hypothesis that genetic variants affecting *TNFRSF11B* predispose to classical PDB.

VCP

The *VCP* gene, encoding valosin-containing protein is known to be the cause of inclusion body myopathy, Paget's disease, and frontotemporal dementia (IBMFPD). Association studies have been conducted to determine if genetic variants of *VCP* contribute to classical PDB. One study in the Belgian and Dutch populations suggests that common variants at the *VCP* locus might predispose to PDB [26] but that was not confirmed in a UK population [27]. Despite this, exome sequencing studies recently identified a novel missense variant in *VCP* which was present in an elderly patient with PDB that did not have any other features of the

IBMPFD syndrome (Albagha and Ralston, unpublished). This is an important finding since it provides proof of concept that rare variants in genes implicated in the rare PDB-like disorders might also be involved in the pathogenesis of PDB.

Chromosome 1p13 Locus

The 1p13 locus was identified as a susceptibility locus for PDB by genome-wide association [12,13]. The associated region extends for approximately 120 kilo bases (kb). The strongest candidate gene is *CSF1* which encodes Macrophage-colony stimulating factor (M-CSF), a key cytokine in the regulation of osteoclast differentiation [28]. Previous studies have shown that rodents with loss of function mutation in *Csf1* gene develop osteopetrosis due to failure of osteoclast differentiation. Additionally, clinical studies have shown that PDB patients have increased serum levels of M-CSF [29], providing further evidence for involvement of *CSF1* in the pathogenesis of PDB. The associated single nucleotide polymorphisms (SNPs) from this region are located upstream *CSF1* and carriers of the risk allele had approximately 70% increased risk of developing PDB. Although it is unclear how SNPs near *CSF1* increase the risk of PDB, it is possible that the identified variants could regulate *CSF1* gene expression directly or indirectly (through linkage disequilibrium with a nearby functional SNP) leading to increased expression of M-CSF and enhanced osteoclast formation. In support of this possibility, the strongest association signal from the GWAS is located in a genomic region rich with histone 3 lysine 27 acetylation (H3K27Ac) harboring several transcription factor binding sites.

Chromosome 7q33

Several SNPs on 7q33 showed strong association with PDB susceptibility in a recent extended GWAS [12]. The associated region is delimited by two recombination hotspots and contains three known genes (*CNOT4*, *NUP205*, and *SLC13A4*). Although any of these could be responsible for the association with PDB due to extensive linkage disequilibrium in the region, the strongest signal was positioned within the *NUP205* gene. This gene encodes a 205 kD nucleoporin protein that forms part of the nuclear pore complex which plays a role in the regulation of transport between the cytoplasm and nucleus. The role of the genes located within this locus in bone metabolism is unknown.

Chromosome 8q24

A genomic region that spans approximately 220 kb on chromosome 8q22 was found to be associated with PDB risk in an extended GWAS [12]. The strongest signal for association clusters within an 18-kb Linkage disequilibrium block spanning the entire *DCSTAMP* gene (also known as Transmembrane 7 superfamily member 4 gene; *TM7SF4*), which encodes dendritic cell-specific transmembrane protein (DC-STAMP). This is a strong functional candidate gene for PDB since it is required for the fusion of osteoclast precursors to form mature osteoclasts [30]. The expression of DC-STAMP is upregulated by RANKL and this molecule is essential for the formation of mature multinucleated osteoclasts [31]. The signaling mechanisms by which DC-STAMP regulates osteoclast precursor fusion are not well-known but a recent study has shown that the connective tissue growth factor CCN2 interacts with DC-STAMP to stimulate osteoclast fusion [32]. It is not yet clear how genetic variants in DC-STAMP lead to increased risk of PDB but since osteoclasts from patients with PDB are larger in size and contain more nuclei than normal osteoclasts, it is possible that these genetic variants predispose to PDB by regulating DC-STAMP expression leading to enhanced osteoclast fusion. This explanation seems likely since the SNP with the strongest association with PDB risk is also an expression quantitative trait locus (eQTL) that was found to regulate the expression of DC-STAMP in peripheral blood monocytes.

Chromosome 10p13

The susceptibility locus for PDB on 10p13 is unusual in that it was found both by linkage in families and by GWAS [13,14]. There is compelling evidence to suggest that the causal gene in 10p13 is *OPTN*. This encodes optineurin which is a widely expressed cytoplasmic protein with multiple cellular functions. Optineurin contains an ubiquitin binding domain similar to that present in NEMO (a component of the IKK complex involved in NFκB signaling pathway). Studies have shown that optineurin negatively regulates TNF-α induced NFκB activation by competing with NEMO for ubiquitylated RIP [33]. Furthermore, a putative NFκB binding site has been identified in *OPTN* promoter and knocking down optineurin by siRNA results in increased basal NFκB activity [34]. Another predicted function of optineurin is in vesicular trafficking between the Golgi apparatus and plasma membrane since it was found to directly interact with myosin VI and Rab 8; both of which have an established role in vesicular trafficking. This is of interest since mutations affecting the VCP protein, which is also involved in vesicular trafficking, cause the syndrome of inclusion body myopathy with early-onset Paget's disease and frontotemporal dementia (IBMPFD) [35].

The causal genetic mutations at this locus have not yet been identified. The predisposing SNP is an extremely strong eQTL for *OPTN* expression in peripheral blood monocytes such that levels of the mRNA are about 15% lower for each susceptibility allele carried [13,36]. Recent functional studies have also shown that mice with a loss of function mutation (D447N) in the ubiquitin binding domain of *Optn* have high bone turnover and that silencing of *Optn* mRNA in bone marrow cultures increases osteoclast formation [36]. The mechanism by which the D447N mutation in *Optn* regulates osteoclast function is complex but it has been shown that the mutated protein is less well able to bind CYLD and that in mutant bone marrow cultures there is enhanced activation of NFκB signaling following RANKL exposure; a reduction in interferon beta production and an increase in *c-fos* expression [36]. Taken together, these data indicate that genetic variants at the 10p13 locus reduce expression of *OPTN*, which predisposes to PDB by activation of NFκB signaling, which, in turn, increases osteoclast differentiation and activity.

Chromosome 14q32

The chromosome 14q32 locus for susceptibility to PDB was identified by an extended GWAS. The region of association extends to 62 kb bound by two recombination hotspots in which is situated the *RIN3* gene, which encodes Ras and Rab interactor 3. The *RIN3* protein is involved in vesicular trafficking to early endosomes and interacts with amphiphysin II, a protein involved in the regulation of endocytosis [37]. It also participates in the internalization of receptor tyrosine kinase KIT in mast cells [38]. Recent studies have shown that *RIN3* is expressed in macrophages and osteoclasts at the mRNA and protein level and although *RIN3* mRNA is also expressed in osteoblasts, the levels are low [39]. At present the mechanisms by which *RIN3* regulates osteoclast activity are unclear but genetic analysis has identified a large number of missense variants within the gene that are overrepresented in PDB cases as compared with controls which are situated throughout the gene product. Most are rare variants but there is one common variant (R279C) predicted to be functional by in silico studies [39]. At the present time it seems likely that the predisposing variants in PDB cause loss of function of *RIN3*, although it is currently unclear which component of *RIN3* function is affected.

Chromosome 15q24

The predisposing region on chromosome 15q24 comprises about 200 kb and was identified by an extended GWAS study. The associated region contains two genes (*PML* and *GOLGA6A*) but SNPs with the highest association signal were clustered within the promyelocytic leukemia gene (*PML*) and the strongest signal was observed for an SNP which results in a phenylalanine to leucine amino acid change at codon 645 (F645L) of the PML protein. The PML protein is involved in a wide range of cellular processes, including apoptosis, tumor suppression, regulation of cell division, differentiation of myeloid precursor cells, and TGF-β signaling. Previous studies have shown that cells from *Pml* knock-out mice are resistant to TGF-β-dependent growth arrest and apoptosis, have impaired induction of TGF-β target genes, and exhibit abnormal nuclear translocation of the TGF-β signaling proteins Smad2 and Smad3 [40]. Since TGF-β is known to play a role in the regulation of bone remodeling, it is possible that the association between PDB and *PML* could be mediated by an effect on TGF-β signaling, but further research will be required to investigate this possibility. The *GOLGA6A* gene is also located in the associated region and encodes a protein that belongs to golgin, a family of coiled-coil proteins associated with the Golgi apparatus, and plays a role in membrane fusion and as structural supports. The function of *GOLGA6A* in bone metabolism has not specifically been investigated but mutations in other members of the golgin family have been shown to cause skeletal dysplasias emphasizing that they do play a role in bone metabolism [41,42].

Chromosome 18q21

The chromosome 18q21 locus was identified by genome-wide association study as predisposing to classical PDB [13], although this locus was also identified by linkage analysis as a predisposing region for familial expansile osteolysis and early onset familial PDB [7,43,44]. The strongest candidate gene in the 18q21 locus is *TNFRSF11A* which encodes receptor activator of NFκB (RANK), a protein that plays a critical role in osteoclast differentiation and activity [45]. Two common SNPs located downstream of

TNFRSF11A were associated with approximately 50% increased risk of PDB in the recent GWAS [13] and several SNPs at the *TNFRSF11A* locus were associated with PDB risk in a candidate gene association study of PDB patients from Belgium, UK, and the Netherlands [46]. The causal genetic variants that predispose to PDB in this region have not yet been identified. The insertion mutations affecting the first exon of *TNFRSF11A*, which cause the syndromes of familial expansile osteolysis, early onset familial PDB, and expansile skeletal hyperphosphatasia, have not been detected in patients with classical PDB disease [47]. Two nonsynonymous polymorphisms have been described in *TNFRSF11A* that cause a histidine to tyrosine amino acid change at codon 141 (H141Y) and a valine to alanine change at codon 192 (V192A). In one report, functional studies were conducted to determine if alleles at the V192A site differed in their ability to activate NFκB in reporter assays. This analysis showed no difference between the ability of alleles to activate NFκB except when they were cotransfected with a *SQSTM1* expression vector when the 192A variant gave greater stimulation of NFκB than the A92V variant [48]. In another study, neither variant was associated with an alteration in NFκB signaling in reporter assays [46].

GENETIC DETERMINANTS OF DISEASE SEVERITY

The clinical presentation and range of complications in PDB vary widely between patients. Whilst, this variation in disease severity can be attributed to genetic factors and/or environmental triggers, studies on the contribution of environmental factors are limited. However, genetic factors have been shown to contribute to the severity of PDB. The clinical presentation of the disease in *SQSTM1* mutation carriers is significantly more severe than noncarriers, with an earlier age at diagnosis and a greater number of affected bones [49]. Moreover, common genetic variants from the seven genetic loci that were identified by GWAS were also associated with disease extent and severity of complications in a recent meta-analysis involving subjects from Italy, UK, Spain, and Western Australia [50]. In this study, patients carrying the greatest number of risk alleles had more extensive disease and had more complications when compared to patients carrying fewer risk alleles, although the effect size of *SQSTM1* mutations was substantially greater than that of the alleles detected by GWAS.

CLINICAL IMPLICATIONS

Genetic studies of PDB have highlighted many new pathways that have not been previously known as players in the regulation of bone metabolism, resulting in major advancements in the understanding of the pathophysiology of the disease. The genetic variants identified from the GWAS study showed a large effect size on PDB risk compared to those observed in many common complex diseases. The combined effect of the seven loci was reported to explain about 13% of the population attributable risk of PDB [12]. The risk of developing PDB was found to increase with the number of risk alleles carried so that patients in the top 10% of the risk allele score distribution have a 10-fold increased risk of having PDB compared to those in the bottom 10%. Once the causal functional variants have been identified from each locus, it is likely that they would have a larger effect size on predicting both disease risk and severity, making them a potentially useful tool in predicting disease risk and complication and in managing treatments. This would be particularly beneficial in PDB which is often diagnosed when complications have already developed and irreversible skeletal damage has occurred [1].

REFERENCES

[1] Tan A, Ralston SH. Clinical presentation of Paget's disease: evaluation of a contemporary cohort and systematic review. Calcif Tissue Int 2014;95(5):385–92.

[2] van Staa TP, Selby P, Leufkens HG, Lyles K, Sprafka JM, Cooper C. Incidence and natural history of Paget's disease of bone in England and Wales. J Bone Miner Res 2002;17(3):465–71.

[3] Montagu MF. Paget's disease (osteitis deformans) and hereditary. Am J Hum Genet 1949;1(1):94–5.

[4] Sofaer JA, Holloway SM, Emery AE. A family study of Paget's disease of bone. J Epidemiol Community Health 1983;37:226–31.

[5] Siris ES, Ottman R, Flaster E, Kelsey JL. Familial aggregation of Paget's disease of bone. J Bone Miner Res 1991;6:495–500.

[6] Morales-Piga AA, Rey-Rey JS, Corres-Gonzalez J, Garcia-Sagredo JM, Lopez-Abente G. Frequency and characteristics of familial aggregation of Paget's disease of bone. J Bone Miner Res 1995;10:663–70.

[7] Hocking L, Slee F, Haslam SI, Cundy T, Nicholson G, Van HW, et al. Familial Paget's disease of bone: patterns of inheritance and frequency of linkage to chromosome 18q. Bone 2000;26(6):577–80.

[8] Laurin N, Brown JP, Lemainque A, Duchesne A, Huot D, Lacourciere Y, et al. Paget disease of bone: mapping of two loci at 5q35-qter and 5q31. Am J Hum Genet 2001;69(3):528–43.

[9] Hocking LJ, Herbert CA, Nicholls RK, Williams F, Bennett ST, Cundy T, et al. Genomewide search in familial paget disease of bone shows evidence of genetic heterogeneity with candidate loci on chromosomes 2q36, 10p13, and 5q35. Am J Hum Genet 2001;69(5):1055–61.

[10] Laurin N, Brown JP, Morissette J, Raymond V. Recurrent mutation of the gene encoding sequestosome 1 (SQSTM1/p62) in Paget disease of bone. Am J Hum Genet 2002;70(6):1582–8.
[11] Hocking LJ, Lucas GJA, Daroszewska A, Mangion J, Olavesen M, Nicholson GC, et al. Domain specific mutations in Sequestosome 1 (SQSTM1) cause familial and sporadic Paget's disease. Hum Mol Genet 2002;11(22):2735–9.
[12] Albagha OME, Wani S, Visconti MR, Alonso N, Goodman K, Cundy T, et al. Genome-wide association identifies three new susceptibility loci for Paget's disease of bone. Nat Genet 2011;43(7):685–9.
[13] Albagha OM, Visconti MR, Alonso N, Langston AL, Cundy T, Dargie R, et al. Genome-wide association study identifies variants at CSF1, OPTN and TNFRSF11A as genetic risk factors for Paget's disease of bone. Nat Genet 2010;42:520–4.
[14] Lucas G, Riches P, Hocking L, Cundy T, Nicholson G, Walsh J, et al. Identification of a major locus for Paget disease on chromosome 10p13 in families of British descent. J Bone Miner Res 2008;23(1):58–63.
[15] Goode A, Long JE, Shaw B, Ralston SH, Visconti MR, Gianfrancesco F, et al. Paget disease of bone-associated UBA domain mutations of SQSTM1 exert distinct effects on protein structure and function. Biochim Biophys Acta 2014;1842 (7):992–1000.
[16] Wright T, Rea SL, Goode A, Bennett AJ, Ratajczak T, Long JE, et al. The S349T mutation of SQSTM1 links Keap1/Nrf2 signalling to Paget's disease of bone. Bone 2013;52(2):699–706.
[17] Sundaram K, Shanmugarajan S, Rao DS, Reddy SV. Mutant p62P392L stimulation of osteoclast differentiation in Paget's disease of bone. Endocrinology 2011;152 (11):4180–9.
[18] Jin W, Chang M, Paul EM, Babu G, Lee AJ, Reiley W, et al. Deubiquitinating enzyme CYLD negatively regulates RANK signaling and osteoclastogenesis in mice. J Clin Invest 2008;118:1858–66.
[19] Chamoux E, Couture J, Bisson M, Morissette J, Brown JP, Roux S. The p62 P392L mutation linked to Paget's disease induces activation of human osteoclasts. Mol Endocrinol 2009;23(10):1668–80.
[20] Simonet WS, Lacey DL, Dunstan CR, Kelley M, Chang MS, Luthy R, et al. Osteoprotegerin: a novel secreted protein involved in the regulation of bone density [see comments]. Cell 1997;89(2):309–19.
[21] Lacey DL, Timms E, Tan HL, Kelley MJ, Dunstan CR, Burgess T, et al. Osteoprotegerin ligand is a cytokine that regulates osteoclast differentiation and activation. Cell 1998;93(2):165–76.
[22] Whyte MP, Obrecht SE, Finnegan PM, Jones JL, Podgornik MN, McAlister WH, et al. Osteoprotegerin deficiency and juvenile Paget's disease. N Engl J Med 2002;347(3):175–84.
[23] Middleton-Hardie C, Zhu Q, Cundy H, Lin JM, Callon K, Tong PC, et al. Deletion of aspartate 182 in OPG causes juvenile Paget's disease by impairing both protein secretion and binding to RANKL. J Bone Miner Res 2006 March;21(3):438–45.
[24] Daroszewska A, Hocking LJ, McGuigan FEA, Langdahl BL, Stone MD, Cundy T, et al. Susceptibility to Paget's disease of bone is influenced by a common polymorphic variant of Osteoprotegerin. J Bone Miner Res 2004;19(9):1506–11.
[25] Beyens G, Daroszewska A, de FF, Fransen E, Vanhoenacker F, Verbruggen L, et al. Identification of sex-specific associations between polymorphisms of the osteoprotegerin gene, TNFRSF11B, and Paget's disease of bone. J Bone Miner Res 2007 July;22(7):1062–71.

[26] Chung PY, Beyens G, de FF, Boonen S, Geusens P, Vanhoenacker F, et al. Indications for a genetic association of a VCP polymorphism with the pathogenesis of sporadic Paget's disease of bone, but not for TNFSF11 (RANKL) and IL-6 polymorphisms. Mol Genet Metab 2011;103(3):287–92.
[27] Lucas GJ, Mehta SG, Hocking LJ, Stewart TL, Cundy T, Nicholson GC, et al. Evaluation of the role of Valosin-containing protein in the pathogenesis of familial and sporadic Paget's disease of bone. Bone 2006;38(2):280–5.
[28] Tanaka S, Takahashi N, Udagawa N, Tamura T, Akatsu T, Stanley ER, et al. Macrophage colony-stimulating factor is indispensable for both proliferation and differentiation of osteoclast progenitors. J Clin Invest 1993;91(1):257–63.
[29] Neale SD, Schulze E, Smith R, Athanasou NA. The influence of serum cytokines and growth factors on osteoclast formation in Paget's disease. QJM 2002;95 (4):233–40.
[30] Yagi M, Miyamoto T, Sawatani Y, Iwamoto K, Hosogane N, Fujita N, et al. DC-STAMP is essential for cell-cell fusion in osteoclasts and foreign body giant cells. J Exp Med 2005;202(3):345–51.
[31] Mensah KA, Ritchlin CT, Schwarz EM. RANKL induces heterogeneous DC-STAMP(lo) and DC-STAMP(hi) osteoclast precursors of which the DC-STAMP(lo) precursors are the master fusogens. J Cell Physiol 2010;223(1):76–83.
[32] Nishida T, Emura K, Kubota S, Lyons KM, Takigawa M. CCN family 2/connective tissue growth factor (CCN2/CTGF) promotes osteoclastogenesis via induction of and interaction with dendritic cell-specific transmembrane protein (DC-STAMP). J Bone Miner Res 2010.
[33] Sudhakar C, Nagabhushana A, Jain N, Swarup G. NF-kappaB mediates tumor necrosis factor alpha-induced expression of optineurin, a negative regulator of NF-kappaB. PLoS One 2009;4(4):e5114.
[34] Zhu G, Wu CJ, Zhao Y, Ashwell JD. Optineurin negatively regulates TNFalpha-induced NF-kappaB activation by competing with NEMO for ubiquitinated RIP. Curr Biol 2007;17(16):1438–43.
[35] Watts GD, Wymer J, Kovach MJ, Mehta SG, Mumm S, Darvish D, et al. Inclusion body myopathy associated with Paget disease of bone and frontotemporal dementia is caused by mutant valosin-containing protein. Nat Genet 2004;36(4):377–81.
[36] Obaid R, Wani S, Ross R, Cohen P, Ralston SH, Albagha OME. Optineurin is a negative regulator of osteoclast differentiation. Cell Reports 2015;13(6):1096–102.
[37] Kajiho H, Saito K, Tsujita K, Kontani K, Araki Y, Kurosu H, et al. RIN3: a novel Rab5 GEF interacting with amphiphysin II involved in the early endocytic pathway. J Cell Sci 2003;116(20):4159–68.
[38] Janson C, Kasahara N, Prendergast GC, Colicelli J. RIN3 is a negative regulator of mast cell responses to SCF. Plos One 2012;7(11):e49615.
[39] Vallet M, Soares DC, Wani S, Sophocleous A, Warner J, Salter DM, et al. Targeted sequencing of the Paget's disease associated 14q32 locus identifies several missense coding variants in RIN3 that predispose to Paget's disease of bone. Hum Mol Genet 2015;24(11):3286–95.
[40] Lin HK, Bergmann S, Pandolfi PP. Cytoplasmic PML function in TGF-beta signalling. Nature 2004;431(7005):205–11.
[41] Hennies HC, Kornak U, Zhang H, Egerer J, Zhang X, Seifert W, et al. Gerodermia osteodysplastica is caused by mutations in SCYL1BP1, a Rab-6 interacting golgin. Nat Genet 2008;40(12):1410–12.
[42] Smits P, Bolton AD, Funari V, Hong M, Boyden ED, Lu L, et al. Lethal skeletal dysplasia in mice and humans lacking the golgin GMAP-210. N Engl J Med 2010;362 (3):206–16.

[43] Haslam SI, Van Hul W, Morales-Piga A, Balemans W, San Millan JL, Nakatsuka K, et al. Paget's disease of bone: evidence for a susceptibility locus on chromosome 18q and for genetic heterogeneity. J Bone Miner Res 1998;13(6):911−17.

[44] Hughes AE, Shearman AM, Weber JL, Barr RJ, Wallace RG, Osterberg PH, et al. Genetic linkage of familial expansile osteolysis to chromosome 18q. Hum Mol Genet 1994;3(2):359−61.

[45] Khosla S. Minireview: the OPG/RANKL/RANK System. Endocrinology 2001;142 (12):5050−5.

[46] Chung PY, Beyens G, Riches PL, Van WL, de FF, Jennes K, et al. Genetic variation in the TNFRSF11A gene encoding RANK is associated with susceptibility to Paget's disease of bone. J Bone Miner Res 2010;25:2316−29.

[47] Sparks AB, Peterson SN, Bell C, Loftus BJ, Hocking L, Cahill DP, et al. Mutation screening of the TNFRSF11A gene encoding receptor activator of NF kappa B (RANK) in familial and sporadic Paget's disease of bone and osteosarcoma. Calcif Tissue Int 2001;68(3):151−5.

[48] Gianfrancesco F, Rendina D, Di SM, Mingione A, Esposito T, Merlotti D, et al. A nonsynonymous TNFRSF11A variation increases NFkappaB activity and the severity of Paget's disease. J Bone Miner Res 2012;27(2):443−52.

[49] Visconti MR, Langston AL, Alonso N, Goodman K, Selby PL, Fraser WD, et al. Mutations of SQSTM1 are associated with severity and clinical outcome in Paget's disease of bone. J Bone Miner Res 2010;25(11):2368−73.

[50] Albagha OM, Visconti MR, Alonso N, Wani S, Goodman K, Fraser WD, et al. Common susceptibility alleles and SQSTM1 mutations predict disease extent and severity in a multinational study of patients with Paget's disease. J Bone Miner Res 2013;28:2238−46.

CHAPTER 4

Developmental Aspects of Pagetic Osteoclasts

Deborah L. Galson[1], Quanhong Sun[1] and G. David Roodman[2,3]
[1]Department of Medicine, Division of Hematology-Oncology, University of Pittsburgh Cancer Institute, University of Pittsburgh School of Medicine, Pittsburgh, PA, United States
[2]Department of Medicine, Division of Hematology-Oncology, Indiana University, Indianapolis, IN, United States
[3]Richard L. Roudebush VA Medical Center, Indianapolis, IN, United States

INTRODUCTION

Paget's disease of bone (PDB) is a complex disease that arises late in life in both patients and in mouse models of PDB. The primary abnormality is in the osteoclast [1], which causes characteristic highly localized bone lesions. The classic description of the pagetic osteoclasts (OCL) phenotype is that there are increased numbers of OCL, that the OCL are unusually large, and have increased numbers of nuclei per OCL. In addition, the pagetic OCL precursors are more sensitive to inducers of OCL formation, such as receptor activator of nuclear factor kappa-B ligand (RANKL), tumor necrosis factor α (TNFα), and 1,25-$(OH)_2D_3$, and form OCL at levels that do not induce normal OCL progenitors to form OCL. The increased bone resorption triggers exuberant bone formation in a coupled response that results in irregular woven bone formation thus yielding weakened bones. A deeper understanding of the molecular alterations in pagetic OCL has provided more detail to the definition of a "pagetic OCL phenotype" that is increasing our understanding of the etiology of PDB.

Both genetic and environmental factors have been implicated in the pathogenesis of PDB [2,4]. Currently, the only gene with protein coding region mutations linked to PDB is sequestosome 1 (*SQSTM1*), which encodes the p62 protein, a scaffold protein that has a key role in cytokine signaling, such as RANKL and TNFα signaling in OCL precursors. Twenty-eight mutations in the *SQSTM1* gene have been identified that all have deleterious effects on ubiquitin binding by p62. The most common mutation, $p62^{P392L}$, is found in 10% of sporadic and 30% of hereditary PDB patients [5–7]. However, mutations in p62 appear insufficient

S.V. Reddy (Ed): Advances in Pathobiology and Management of Paget's Disease of Bone.
DOI: http://dx.doi.org/10.1016/B978-0-12-805083-5.00004-X

to induce PDB since 15–20% of individuals carrying p62 mutations fail to develop the disease [8]. Further, Kurihara and coworkers showed that both transgenic mice expressing human $p62^{P392L}$ specifically in OCL (*TRAP-p62* mice), as well as knockin mice harboring germline $p62^{P394L}$, the murine equivalent of human $p62^{P392L}$, (*p62KI* mice) have increased numbers of OCL precursors and OCL, but the OCL do not have a "pagetic phenotype," nor do the mice develop the bone lesions characteristic of PDB [9,10]. These results show that genetic factors increase OCL numbers, but environmental factors are also required for the increased bone formation characteristic of PDB. Daroszewska et al. [11] also analyzed a $p62^{P394L}$ knockin mouse model and found small pagetic lesions in the long bones, but not in the vertebrae. It is unclear why the two mouse models yielded different results, but suggests that there may have been an additional environmental factor involved.

Recently in PDB patients without *SQSTM1* mutations, increased risk of developing PDB has been linked to susceptibility genetic polymorphisms in regions containing genes for calcium-sensing receptor (*CASR*), estrogen receptor 1 (*ESR1*), osteoprotegerin (OPG; *TNFRSF11B*), RANK (*TNFRSF11A*), macrophage colony stimulating factor (M-CSF; *CSF1*), optineurin (*OPTN*), dendritic-cell-specific transmembrane protein (DC-STAMP; *TM7SF4*), valosin containing protein (*VCP*), nucleoporin 205 kDa (*NUP205*), Ras and Rab interactor 3 (*RIN3*), promyelocytic leukemia (*PML*), and golgin A6 family, member A (*GOLGA6A*) [4]. Many of these genes have known functions in OCL but how the polymorphisms (none of which are in the coding region of these genes) impact the expression and function of these genes on signal transduction events in OCL remains unclear. Also, how they would interact with mutations in p62 and environmental factors has not yet been assessed.

Environmental factors, including measles virus (MV) and other paramyxoviruses, have also been implicated in the pathogenesis of PDB. Pagetic osteoclasts demonstrate the presence of paramyxoviral-like nuclear inclusions. Reddy et al. [12] generated a transgenic mouse expressing the human MV receptor CD46 in the OCL lineage. They found that in vitro MV infection of OCL precursors from these mice generated OCL with many features of pagetic OCL. OCLs from 70% of PDB patients express the measles virus nucleocapsid protein (MVNP) gene, and normal OCL precursors expressing MVNP formed OCLs that exhibit the pagetic phenotype [9,13,14]. In addition MVNP can induce the pagetic OCL phenotype in vitro and in vivo in transgenic mice expressing MVNP in OCL lineage cells (*MVNP* mice) [15]. Most importantly, it was recently reported that antisense knockdown of MVNP in OCL lineage cells in MVNP-positive OCL from PDB patients carrying $p62^{P392L}$ resulted in loss of the pagetic phenotype [9]. Further, when p62KI mice were bred to *MVNP* mice, the *p62KI/MVNP* mice developed greater numbers of pagetic OCL than either genotype alone, and dramatic pagetic bone lesions that were strikingly similar to those seen in patients with PDB [9]. While MVNP is likely not the only environmental factor that contributes to the development of PDB, it is the best proven and characterized.

We will discuss the state of knowledge of the pagetic OCL phenotype and the individual contributions of genetic ($p62^{P392L}$) and environmental (MVNP) factors to these changes (Table 4.1).

Table 4.1 Pagetic OCL phenotype and the contributions of MVNP and $p62^{P392L}$

Characteristics of pagetic OCL	PDB patients	MVNP	$p62^{P392L}$
Hyperresponsive to RANKL & TNFα	+	+	+
Hyperresponsive to $1,25(OH)_2D_3$	+	+	-
Increased OCL numbers in vitro and in vivo	+	+	+
Increased nuclei number/OCL in vitro and in vivo	+	+	-
Increased OCL size in vitro and in vivo	+	+	+
Increased bone resorption/OCL	+	+	-
Increased IL-6 expression	+	+	-
Increased IGF1 expression	+	+	-
Increased FGF2 expression	+	+	?
Increased CXCL5 expression	+	+	-
Increased TBK1 protein level and activity	+	+	-
Decreased OPTN protein level	+	+	-
Decreased Sirt1 expression	?	+	?
Decreased FoxO3 protein level	?	+	?
Increased NFκB expression and activity	+	+	+
Increased NFATc1 expression and activity	+	+	+
Increased TAF12 expression and activity	+	+	-
Increased ATF7 expression and activity	?	+	-
Increased EphrinB2 by mature OCL	+	+	-
Induce increased osteoblast EphB4	+	+	-
Induce increased bone formation in vivo	+	+	-

+, Changed from normal; -, No change from normal; ?, Not known.

INCREASED SENSITIVITY OF OCL PROGENITORS TO OSTEOTROPIC FACTORS

In marrow cultures from PDB patients, OCL precursors form OCL in response to 1,25-$(OH)_2D_3$ at physiological (10^{-12} to 10^{-11} M) concentrations rather than the pharmacological (10^{-8} M) concentration required for OCL formation in marrow cultures from normal subjects [13]. In addition, OCL precursors from PDB have increased sensitivity to RANKL [2,16] and TNFα [10], responding to 10-fold lower concentrations than normal precursors. However, OCL precursors from either *TRAP-p62* or *p62KI* mice are hyperresponsive to RANKL and TNFα, but not to 1,25-$(OH)_2D_3$ [9,10]. In contrast, OCL precursors from *MVNP* mice are hyperresponsive to all three OCL inducers [15]. OCL precursors from PDB patients with $p62^{P293L}$ that were hyperresponsive to 1,25-$(OH)_2D_3$ were found to be MVNP positive, and knockdown of MVNP reduced the 1,25-$(OH)_2D_3$ sensitivity [9].

Increased Sensitivity to RANKL and TNFα

Both RANKL and TNFα activate signaling pathways involving p62, which serves as a platform molecule with multiple protein interaction domains that brings together upstream and downstream signal transducers, that ultimately lead to the activation of the p38 MAPK and ERK1/2 pathways, as well as IκB kinase (IKK) complex (IKKα,β,γ) activation of the transcription factor NFκB, all downstream events that are important for OCL formation and function [17]. The binding of RANKL to its receptor RANK results in the recruitment and activation of TRAF6 via K63-linked ubiquitination [18]. Activated TRAF6 then stimulates activation of the IKK complex via TAB1/TAB2/TAK1-dependent [19] or atypical PKC (aPKC)-dependent phosphorylation [20]. The scaffolding protein p62 is one of the functional links between TRAF6 and activation of the IKK complex [20]. p62 binds both TRAF6 and aPKCs (PKCζ and PKCλ) resulting in the formation of a multimeric protein complex that regulates NFκB activation via phosphorylation of IKKβ [20,21]. Similarly, TNFα interaction with its receptor TNFR1 triggers formation of signal transducing complexes that include the kinase receptor interacting protein 1 (RIP1) bound to p62, which then leads to recruitment of aPKCs and downstream signal activation [22]. However, p62 also functions to attenuate TRAF6 and RIP1 signaling by recruiting the deubiquitinase cylindromatosis (CYLD), via binding to the ubiquitin chains on

CYLD [23]. Loss of p62 binding to ubiquitin chains as a result of pagetic mutations decreases recruitment of CYLD [24], decreasing the signal attenuation and leading to increased signaling at lower ligand-receptor interaction levels (Fig. 4.1). Interestingly, both in transduced human OCL precursors and transgenic mice, p62^{P392L} had a much more dramatic effect increasing the sensitivity to TNFα than to RANKL [9], suggesting that TNFα regulation of OCL formation may be more subject to negative regulation by p62 recruitment of deubiquitinases such as CYLD than RANKL.

MVNP also increases the response of OCL precursors to RANKL and TNFα, but the mechanisms are just beginning to be determined. MVNP has been reported to activate the antiviral response by interacting with a complex containing transcription factor IRF3 and the noncanonical IKK-related homologous kinases, TANK-binding kinase 1 (TBK1) and IKKε [25,26] MVNP activated TBK1 and IKKε phosphorylate IRF3, thereby allowing it to dimerize and translocate into the nucleus to induce IRF3 target genes, such as interferon β (IFNβ). TBK1 and IKKε can also activate NFκB, both by directly phosphorylating NFκB as well as functioning

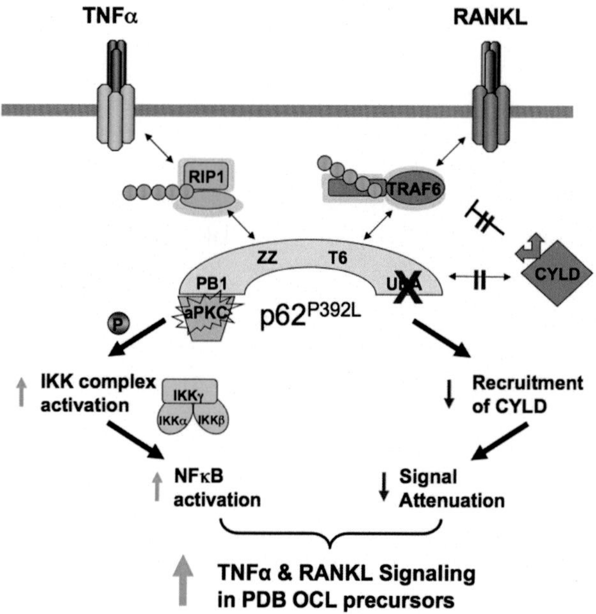

Figure 4.1 Mechanisms by which p62P392L increases cytokine sensitivity in osteoclast precursors.

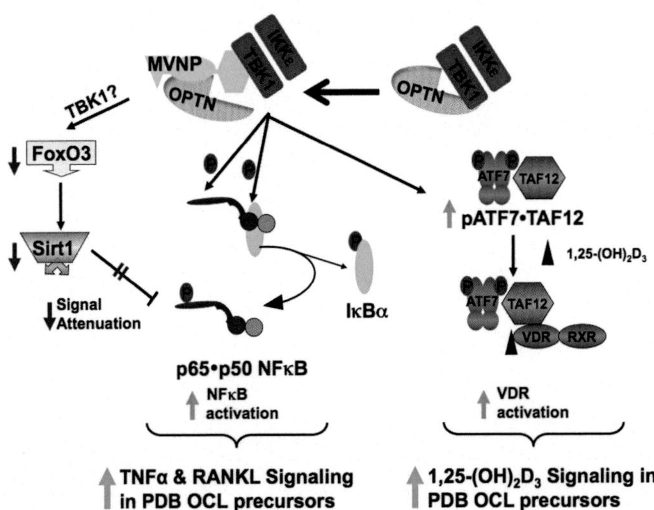

Figure 4.2 Mechanisms by which MVNP increases cytokine and 1,25-(OH)2D3 sensitivity in osteoclast precursors.

upstream of the canonical IKK complex [27–29]. MVNP elevates both total NFκB and phospho-S536-p65 NFκB in OCL precursors, and can increase expression of a NFκB reporter [13,30,31]. Further, Sun et al. [32,33] recently reported that MVNP expression in bone marrow monocytes (BMM) decreased protein levels of optineurin (OPTN), most closely related to IKKγ (also known as NEMO), and demonstrated that OPTN is a novel negative regulator of OCL formation in vitro using OPTN overexpression and knockdown in mouse BMM. OPTN binds TBK1 [34], but its role in regulating TBK1 activity is unclear, with reports of both positive [35] and negative [36] regulation. However, Sun et al. [32,33]. reported that ectopic OPTN blocked MVNP or TBK1 activation of NFκB and interleukin-6 (IL-6) expression. Further, OPTN has been reported to block TNFα activation of NEMO by recruiting CYLD to RIP1, leading to decreased NFκB activity [37,38]. This suggests that MVNP increases the sensitivity of OCL precursors to RANKL and TNFα by lowering the threshold necessary to trigger a response through activating TBK1 and decreasing OPTN (Fig. 4.2).

Increased Sensitivity to 1,25-(OH)$_2$D$_3$

MVNP, but not p62^{P392L}, induces increased sensitivity to 1,25-(OH)$_2$D$_3$ in PDB [9,15,39]. The enhanced sensitivity results from

MVNP-increased expression of transcription initiation factor TFIID subunit 12 (TAF12; formerly known as TAF_{II}-17), a member of the TFIID transcription factor complex. Importantly, TAF12 also functions as a vitamin D receptor (VDR) coactivator in multiple cell types, thereby enhancing the ability of VDR to respond to lower amounts of its ligand 1,25-$(OH)_2D_3$ in MVNP-expressing OCL precursors [40]. Knockdown of TAF12 in OCL precursors from MVNP-expressing *p62*^{P392L} PDB patients with a TAF12 antisense construct decreased the 1,25-$(OH)_2D_3$ sensitivity and OCL formation, but did not affect normal OCL formation [9]. This indicates that TAF12 induced by MVNP contributes to the pagetic OCL phenotype. In addition, overexpression of TAF12 in normal human OCL precursors (by retrovirus infection) or in transgenic mouse OCL precursors (*TRAP-TAF12* mice) demonstrated increased sensitivity to 1,25-$(OH)_2D_3$ and formed OCL at lower levels than wild type cells [41,42]. However, these OCLs failed to exhibit other hallmarks of the pagetic OCL phenotype, such as increased sensitivity to RANKL and hypermultinucleation. Further, the *TRAP-TAF12* mice did not develop pagetic lesions, indicating that increased TAF12 expression and 1,25-$(OH)_2D_3$ signaling may be necessary, but is not sufficient to generate the full pagetic phenotype. TAF12 was found to interact with the bZIP activating transcription factor 7 (ATF7) and potentiate ATF7-driven genes [42]. Coimmunoprecipitation studies revealed that TAF12 interacts with ATF7 in OCL precursors. MVNP expression elevated ATF7 protein levels compared to normal OCL precursors independent of 1,25-$(OH)_2D_3$. Knockdown of ATF7 in MVNP-expressing cells decreased 1,25-$(OH)_2D_3$ induction of a VDR-target gene, cytochrome P450, family 24, subfamily A, polypeptide 1 (*Cyp24A1*) and TAF12 binding to a *Cyp24A1* promoter containing two functionally important VDR binding sites. Thus, ATF7 increases the TAF12 contribution towards hypersensitivity to 1,25-$(OH)_2D_3$ of pagetic OCL precursors (Fig. 4.2).

INCREASED NUCLEI/OCL

Osteoclasts differentiate from precursors in the monocyte-macrophage lineage in response to M-CSF and RANKL. Multinuclear OCL arise from fusion of mononuclear precursor cells. Multinucleation increases the OCL size and enhances the resorbing efficiency of OCL both in vivo and in vitro. Hypermultinucleated OCL are observed in PDB lesions and are increased in both number and size, and in cross-section are seen to contain up to 100 nuclei, in contrast to normal osteoclasts, which contain 3–10 nuclei [2] However, the cellular mechanics controlling OCL size are poorly understood. Several proteins upregulated by RANKL are known to be involved in the fusion process, including DC-STAMP, OC-STAMP, the d2 isoform of the vacuolar ATPase V0 proton pump (Atp6v0d2), and CD9, a member of the transmembrane 4 superfamily [43]. MVNP expressing OCL precursors form hypermultinucleated OCLs, whereas $p62^{P392L}$ does not increase the nuclei number/OCL [9,10,15]. MVNP increases OCL production of IL-6, and IL-6 has been demonstrated to increase the number of nuclei/OCL in the presence of low levels of 1,25-$(OH)_2D_3$ [9]. Also, we [44] and others [45] have observed that MVNP increases both the level and signaling of nuclear factor of activate T cells (NFATc1), a key osteoclast transcription factor that regulates the expression of at least two fusion molecules, DC-STAMP and Atp6v0d2. However, $p62^{P392L}$ has also been reported to elevate NFATc1 [24]. Little is known about the effect of either MVNP or mutant p62 on the RANKL-regulated fusion molecules, DC-STAMP, OC-STAMP, Atp6v0d2, or CD9, or other non-RANKL regulation fusion molecules that are also expressed in OCL, such as CD44, CD47, TREM2 [43]. So, understanding the regulation of this aspect of the pagetic OCL phenotype awaits further study.

INCREASED EXPRESSION OF IL-6

PDB patients have elevated IL-6 levels in their marrow plasma and peripheral blood, and their OCL express high levels of IL-6 [9,46]. A neutralizing antibody to IL-6 blocked the increased OCL formation observed in PDB patient marrow cultures [47] and induced by MV infection of hCD46 + murine bone marrow cultures [12]. Kurihara et al. [9] reported that IL-6 deficiency in *MVNP* mice abrogates the development of pagetic OCL in vitro and in vivo. This demonstrated that expression of MVNP in OCL precursors induces high levels of IL-6 expression that are essential for the formation of pagetic OCL and bone lesions. In contrast, OCL from *p62KI* mice do not express elevated IL-6 levels, nor does the *p62KI* mouse model produce pagetic lesions in the absence of MVNP [9]. These results suggest that IL-6 plays a key role in the effects of MVNP on OCL activity in PDB. However, Teramachi et al. [48] recently showed that increased IL-6 expression in osteoclasts is necessary but not sufficient for the development of PDB.

Hence, the regulation of IL-6 expression by MVNP is of importance in understanding the mechanisms by which MVNP contributes to aberrant OCL formation in PDB. MVNP increases *IL-6* gene transcription, while *IL-6* mRNA stability remains unchanged [31]. While an array of transcription factors have been reported to regulate *IL-6* in response to different stimuli in a variety of cell types, the studies indicate that NFκB is important for basal *IL-6* expression [49]. Transfection studies have demonstrated that while NFκB is important for both basal and for part of the MVNP-stimulation of *IL-6* expression, there is an additional factor that makes a significant contribution to MVNP-induced *IL-6* expression. Among the transcription factors known to synergize with NFκB to activate the *IL-6* gene promoter is the bZIP transcription factor C/EBPβ The authors have shown that MVNP increases C/EBPβ and used chromatin immunoprecipitation to reveal that MVNP increases both NFκB and C/EBPβ occupancy on the endogenous *IL-6* gene promoter in NIH3T3 cells (unpublished data).

MVNP Activation of TBK1 Increases IL-6, OCL Formation, and Nuclei/OCL

Sun et al. [30] reported that MVNP increases TBK1 in BMM by increasing TBK1 protein stability resulting in increased phosphorylated active TBK1 present. Similar to MVNP expression, TBK1 overexpression in several cell lines increased *IL-6*-promoter reporter activity, endogenous *IL-6* mRNA, activated p65 NFκB, as well as TAF12 and ATF7 proteins. Overexpression of TAF12 in OCL progenitors from TRAP-TAF12 mice not only were hypersensitive to 1,25-$(OH)_2D_3$ as mentioned above, but also produced increased levels of IL-6 compared to wild type cells [41,42]. This suggests that TBK1 might regulate the *IL-6* gene through inducing increased NFκB, C/EBPβ and TAF12, although it is not yet known by what mechanism TAF12 regulates *IL-6*. Ectopic TBK1 (via lentiviral transduction) or in transgenic mouse OCL precursors (*TRAP-TBK1* mice) in vitro was sufficient to induce pagetic OCL formation in response to RANKL, including increased IL-6, OCL formation, and nuclei/OCL [32,33]. Pharmaceutical inhibition of both TBK1 and its homolog IKKε with BX795 or amlexanox impaired MVNP-induced IL-6 expression in NIH3T3 cells and in BMM from MVNP mice, and decreased OCL formation. Further, knockdown of TBK1 in *MVNP* BMM specifically impaired development of the MVNP-induced pagetic OCL phenotype. Hence, TBK1 plays a critical role in mediating the effects of MVNP on IL-6 expression and OCL differentiation (Fig. 4.2) [30,32,33].

MVNP Downregulation of FoxO3 and Sirt1 also Increase IL-6

MVNP also was demonstrated to increase NFκB activity by downregulating expression of Sirtuin 1 (Sirt1), a class III protein deacetylase that targets acetylated NFκB and negatively regulates its activity [31]. MVNP decreases Sirt1 by triggering increased phosphorylation of Forkhead-box class O3 (FoxO3), resulting in decreased FoxO3 protein stability and decreased transcription of its target gene *Sirt1* in OCL precursors and NIH3T3 cells. Several protein kinases have been reported to downregulate FoxO3 stability through phosphorylation, including AKT, ERK1/2, IKKβ, and IKKε [50–52]. It's not yet known which, if any, of these are triggered by MVNP to phosphorylate FoxO3. However, TBK1 overexpression in *TRAP-TBK1* BMM was sufficient to decrease Sirt1 mRNA (unpublished data), suggesting that activated TBK1 may phosphorylate FoxO3. Wang et al. [31] showed that NIH3T3 cells stably transduced with MVNP (MVNP-NIH3T3) demonstrated higher *IL-6* promoter luciferase reporter activity than NIH3T3 cells transduced with empty vector (EV-NIH3T3), and ectopic expression of Sirt1 significantly decreased both the basal and MVNP-stimulated *IL-6* promoter activity. Further, resveratrol, a *Sirt1* gene activator, suppressed the high level of *IL-6* mRNA in MVNP-NIH3T3 cells. Significantly, resveratrol inhibited OCL differentiation of BMM from both wild-type and *MVNP* mice. Strikingly, at a resveratrol dose that had little effect on wild-type OCL differentiation, the enhanced *MVNP* OCL differentiation was suppressed to wild-type levels. Higher resveratrol doses then suppressed wild-type and *MVNP* OCL differentiation to similar levels. Hence, MVNP acts via two pathways to increase *IL-6* expression (Fig. 4.2).

INCREASED IRREGULAR WOVEN BONE FORMATION INDUCED BY PAGETIC OCL

Bone resorption and bone formation are tightly linked processes, with bone formation normally occurring only at sites of previous bone resorption. PDB represents the most exaggerated example of coupled bone remodeling in which both OCL and osteoblast activity is markedly increased. This results in rapid focal overproduction of bone that is of poor quality and can cause significant clinical problems for PDB patients, including bone deformity, fracture, secondary osteoarthritis in joints between pagetic lesions, skull thickening, and nerve compression syndromes. The OCLs in PDB play a critical role in the enhanced osteoblast activity observed in these patients since therapies that decrease OCL activity also decrease new bone formation and induce clinical remission in PDB [53].

EphrinB2/EphB4 Signaling

EphrinB2 expressed by OCL and EphB4 expressed by osteoblasts were recently identified as key coupling factors whose interaction stimulates bone formation and inhibits OCL activity [54]. Teramachi and coworkers [3,55,56] recently reported that EphrinB2/EphB4 was increased in bone marrow cultures from aged *MVNP* mice (8–12 month old) as compared to WT, *TRAP-p62*, and *p62KI* mice. This is consistent with the observation that only mice 8 months or older develop pagetic lesions [9,11,15]. Interestingly, the effects of MVNP on EphrinB2 expression by OCL lineage cells in response to 1,25-$(OH)_2D_3$ were biphasic, with early *MVNP* OCL precursors (CD11b + cells) expressing lower levels than WT OCL, whereas more differentiated *MVNP* OCL expressed higher levels than WT, *TRAP-p62*, and *p62KI* OCL. Further, 1,25-$(OH)_2D_3$-treated osteoblasts derived from bone marrow cultures from *MVNP* mice had increased expression of EphB4 and Runx2 as compared to WT and *TRAP-p62* mice. They found that OCL from *MVNP* mice express elevated ephrinB2 as a result of the increased IL-6 and that this contributes to the increased bone formation. *MVNP* mice with IL-6 deficiency had decreased expression of EphrinB2, EphB4 and Runx2, consistent with the lack of increased bone formation in these mice. These results suggest that MVNP promotes coupled bone formation via an IL-6-dependent mechanism that increases EphrinB2 and EphB4 on OCL and osteoblasts, respectively, thereby increasing EphrinB2-EphB4 signaling (Fig. 4.3).

IGF1, FGF2, and CXCL5

Teramachi and coworkers [55,56] also reported that insulin-like growth factor 1 (IGF1), which has a role in increasing bone matrix mineralization [57], is elevated in OCL precursors from *MVNP* mice relative to WT and *p62KI* mice, and may regulate the expression of OCL EphrinB2 and osteoblast EphB4. The enhanced IL-6 expression played a role in the elevated IGF1 levels produced by pagetic OCL, and together IL-6 and IGF1

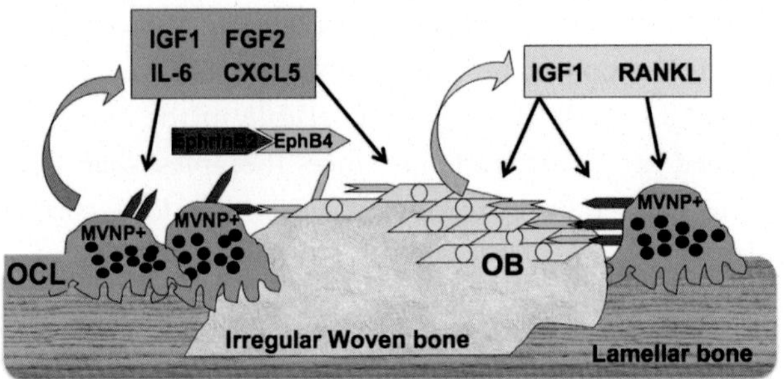

Figure 4.3 MVNP increases OCL induction of osteoblast differentiation.

are major contributors to the rapid bone formation in PDB. Interestingly fibroblast growth factor 2 (FGF2) was reported to be elevated in the serum of PDB patients and increased by MVNP expression in OCL precursors [58], and FGF2 was reported to elevate osteoblast expression of IGF1 [59], which may then add to the MVNP-induced OCL production of IGF1 to increase bone formation. These authors also reported that FGF2 increased stromal cell production of RANKL, thereby completing the feedback loop to increase OCL formation. Sundaram et al. [60] recently identified that both chemokine (C-X-C motif) ligand 5 (CXCL5) mRNA expression and serum protein levels were significantly increased in patients with PDB compared with that in normal subjects, and increased by MVNP expression in OCL precursors. Increased CXCL5 also increases stromal cell production of RANKL, thereby, further enhancing OCL formation.

CONCLUSION

The scaffold protein p62 protein has specific interaction domains for both RIP1 (ZZ domain) and TRAF6 (T6), as well as an N-terminal domain that binds aPKC (PB1) and a C-terminal ubiquitin associated domain (UBA). There are also other domains and interactions not discussed in this chapter. Interaction of the cytokines RANKL and TNFα with their respective receptors, RANK and TNFR1, activates TRAF6 and RIP1, respectively, by inducing K63-linked ubiquitination. TRAF6 and RIP1 are bound by p62, which both activates downstream signaling by recruiting and activating aPKC to phosphorylate IKKβ, and attenuates the RANKL and TNFα signaling by recruiting the deubiquitinase CYLD via the p62 UBD to deubiquinate TRAF6 and RIP1. However, $p62^{P392L}$ has a defective UBD and does not recruit CYLD, thereby decreasing attenuation of the RANKL and TNFα signals resulting in increased cytokine signaling.

MVNP interaction with the TBK1-OPTN complex prevents OPTN from inhibiting TBK1, thereby increasing activated TBK1, which results in direct phosphorylation of S536-p65 NFκB, leading to increased activation and nuclear translocation of NFκB. MNVP interaction with OPTN leads to decreased OPTN, thereby also decreasing attenuation of TNFα induction of NFκB activation. MVNP activation of an unknown kinase, which may be TBK1, leads to phosphorylation and degradation of FoxO3, leading to decreased expression of its target gene, *Sirt1*, which attenuates NFκB activity by deacetylating NFκB. Thus, MVNP induces both increased activation and decreased attenuation of NFκB, thereby increasing the response to the cytokines RANKL and TNFα. TBK1 activity also stimulates increased ATF7 activation and increased TAF12 levels, thereby enhancing the sensitivity of VDR to 1,25-$(OH)_2D_3$.

MVNP expression in PDB OCL results in secretion of high levels of IL-6 and IGF (pink box) that act on OCL to induce increased expression of EphrinB2 and act on osteoblasts (OB) to increase expression of EphB4. The enhanced interaction of EphrinB2 and EphB4 leads to increased coupled bone formation. Further, MVNP enhances OCL production of FGF2 and CXCL5 (pink box), which act on OB lineage cells to increase RANKL (blue box) production, producing a positive feedback loop to further enhance OCL formation. In addition, FGF2 increases osteoblast production of IGF1 (blue box), which acts together with the OCL produced IGF1 (pink box) to increase bone formation.

Disclosures

GD Roodman is on the Advisory Board of Amgen. GD Roodman received grant NIAMS/NIH R01 AR57308 and Research Funds from the Veteran's Administration. DL Galson received grant NIAMS/NIH R01 AR57310.

REFERENCES

[1] Rebel A, Malkani K, Basle M, Bregeon C. Osteoclast ultrastructure in Paget's disease. Calcif Tissue Res 1976;2:187–99.
[2] Roodman GD, Windle JJ. Paget disease of bone. J Clin Invest 2005;115(2):200–8.
[3] Teramachi J, Kurihara N, Windle JJ, Roodman GD. Expression of measles virus nucleocapsid protein (MVNP) gene in osteoclasts induces coupling factors that stimulate bone formation. J Bone Miner Res 2012;27(Suppl. 1):S497.

[4] Chung PY, Van Hul W. Paget's disease of bone: evidence for complex pathogenetic interactions. Semin Arthritis Rheum 2012;41(5):619–41.
[5] Hocking LJ, Lucas GJ, Daroszewska A, et al. Domain-specific mutations in sequestosome 1 (SQSTM1) cause familial and sporadic Paget's disease. Hum Mol Genet 2002;11(22):2735–9.
[6] Laurin N, Brown JP, Morissette J, Raymond V. Recurrent mutation of the gene encoding sequestosome 1 (SQSTM1/p62) in Paget disease of bone. Am J Hum Genet 2002;70(6):1582–8.
[7] Morissette J, Laurin N, Brown JP. Sequestosome 1: mutation frequencies, haplotypes, and phenotypes in familial Paget's disease of bone. J Bone Miner Res 2006;21 (Suppl 2):38–44.
[8] Rea SL, Walsh JP, Layfield R, Ratajczak T, Xu J. New insights into the role of sequestosome 1/p62 mutant proteins in the pathogenesis of Paget's disease of bone. Endocr Rev 2013;34(4):501–24.
[9] Kurihara N, Hiruma Y, Yamana K, et al. Contributions of the measles virus nucleocapsid gene and the SQSTM1/p62(P392L) mutation to Paget's disease. Cell Metab 2011;13(1):23–34.
[10] Kurihara N, Hiruma Y, Zhou H, et al. Mutation of the sequestosome 1 (p62) gene increases osteoclastogenesis but does not induce Paget disease. J Clin Invest 2007;117 (1):133–42.
[11] Daroszewska A, van 't Hof RJ, Rojas JA, et al. A point mutation in the ubiquitin-associated domain of SQSMT1 is sufficient to cause a Paget's disease-like disorder in mice. Hum Mol Genet 2011;20(14):2734–44.
[12] Reddy SV, Kurihara N, Menaa C, et al. Osteoclasts formed by measles virus-infected osteoclast precursors from hCD46 transgenic mice express characteristics of pagetic osteoclasts. Endocrinology 2001;142(7):2898–905.
[13] Kurihara N, Reddy SV, Menaa C, Anderson D, Roodman GD. Osteoclasts expressing the measles virus nucleocapsid gene display a pagetic phenotype. J Clin Invest 2000;105(5):607–14.
[14] Reddy SV, Singer FR, Roodman GD. Bone marrow mononuclear cells from patients with Paget's disease contain measles virus nucleocapsid messenger ribonucleic acid that has mutations in a specific region of the sequence. J Clin Endocrinol Metab 1995;80(7):2108–11.
[15] Kurihara N, Zhou H, Reddy SV, et al. Expression of measles virus nucleocapsid protein in osteoclasts induces Paget's disease-like bone lesions in mice. J Bone Miner Res 2006;21(3):446–55.
[16] Neale SD, Smith R, Wass JA, Athanasou NA. Osteoclast differentiation from circulating mononuclear precursors in Paget's disease is hypersensitive to 1,25-dihydroxyvitamin D(3) and RANKL. Bone 2000;27(3):409–16.
[17] Roodman GD. Insights into the pathogenesis of Paget's disease. Ann N Y Acad Sci 2010;1192:176–80.
[18] Ye H, Arron JR, Lamothe B, et al. Distinct molecular mechanism for initiating TRAF6 signalling. Nature 2002;418(6896):443–7.
[19] Besse A, Lamothe B, Campos AD, et al. TAK1-dependent signaling requires functional interaction with TAB2/TAB3. J Biol Chem 2007;282(6):3918–28.
[20] Duran A, Serrano M, Leitges M, et al. The atypical PKC-interacting protein p62 is an important mediator of RANK-activated osteoclastogenesis. Dev Cell 2004;6 (2):303–9.
[21] Chamoux E, McManus S, Laberge G, Bisson M, Roux S. Involvement of kinase PKC-zeta in the p62/p62(P392L)-driven activation of NF-kappaB in human osteoclasts. Biochim Biophys Acta 2013;1832(3):475–84.

[22] Sanz L, Sanchez P, Lallena MJ, Diaz-Meco MT, Moscat J. The interaction of p62 with RIP links the atypical PKCs to NF-kappaB activation. Embo J 1999;18 (11):3044–53.
[23] Jin W, Chang M, Paul EM, et al. Deubiquitinating enzyme CYLD negatively regulates RANK signaling and osteoclastogenesis in mice. J Clin Invest 2008;118 (5):1858–66.
[24] Sundaram K, Shanmugarajan S, Rao DS, Reddy SV. Mutant p62P392L stimulation of osteoclast differentiation in Paget's disease of bone. Endocrinology 2011;152 (11):4180–9.
[25] Fitzgerald KA, McWhirter SM, Faia KL, et al. IKKepsilon and TBK1 are essential components of the IRF3 signaling pathway. Nat Immunol 2003;4(5):491–6.
[26] Sharma S, tenOever BR, Grandvaux N, Zhou GP, Lin R, Hiscott J. Triggering the interferon antiviral response through an IKK-related pathway. Science 2003;300 (5622):1148–51.
[27] Buss H, Dorrie A, Schmitz ML, Hoffmann E, Resch K, Kracht M. Constitutive and interleukin-1-inducible phosphorylation of p65 NF-κB at serine 536 is mediated by multiple protein kinases including IκB kinase (IKK)-α, IKKβ, IKKε, TRAF family member-associated (TANK)-binding kinase 1 (TBK1), and an unknown kinase and couples p65 to TATA-binding protein-associated factor II31-mediated interleukin-8 transcription. J Biol Chem 2004;279(53):55633–43.
[28] Nomura F, Kawai T, Nakanishi K, Akira S. NF-kappaB activation through IKK-i-dependent I-TRAF/TANK phosphorylation. Genes Cells 2000;5(3):191–202.
[29] Pomerantz JL, Baltimore D. NF-kappaB activation by a signaling complex containing TRAF2, TANK and TBK1, a novel IKK-related kinase. Embo J 1999;18 (23):6694–704.
[30] Sun Q, Sammut B, Wang FM, et al. TBK1 mediates critical effects of measles virus nucleocapsid protein (MVNP) on pagetic osteoclast formation. J Bone Miner Res 2014;29(1):90–102.
[31] Wang FM, Sarmasik A, Hiruma Y, et al. Measles virus nucleocapsid protein, a key contributor to Paget's disease, increases IL-6 expression via down-regulation of FoxO3/Sirt1 signaling. Bone 2013;53(1):269–76.
[32] Sun Q, Adamik J, Windle JJ, Roodman GD, Galson DL. Decreased optineurin mediates MVNP effects in pagetic osteoclasts. J Bone Miner Res 2014;29(Suppl 1).
[33] Sun Q, Zhang P, Adamik J, et al. MVNP alters the balance of TBK1 and optineurin in osteoclast lineage cells to generate pagetic osteoclasts. J Bone Miner Res 2015;30 (Suppl 1):S333.
[34] Morton S, Hesson L, Peggie M, Cohen P. Enhanced binding of TBK1 by an optineurin mutant that causes a familial form of primary open angle glaucoma. FEBS Lett 2008;582(6):997–1002.
[35] Gleason CE, Ordureau A, Gourlay R, Arthur JS, Cohen P. Polyubiquitin binding to optineurin is required for optimal activation of TANK-binding kinase 1 and production of interferon beta. J Biol Chem 2011;286(41):35663–74.
[36] Mankouri J, Fragkoudis R, Richards KH, et al. Optineurin negatively regulates the induction of IFNbeta in response to RNA virus infection. PLoS Pathog 2010;6(2): e1000778.
[37] Nagabhushana A, Bansal M, Swarup G. Optineurin is required for CYLD-dependent inhibition of TNFalpha-induced NF-kappaB activation. PLoS One 2011;6(3):e17477.
[38] Zhu G, Wu CJ, Zhao Y, Ashwell JD. Optineurin negatively regulates TNFalpha-induced NF-kappaB activation by competing with NEMO for ubiquitinated RIP. Curr Biol 2007;17(16):1438–43.

[39] Hiruma Y, Kurihara N, Subler MA, et al. A SQSTM1/p62 mutation linked to Paget's disease increases the osteoclastogenic potential of the bone microenvironment. Hum Mol Genet 2008;17(23):3708–19.
[40] Mengus G, Gangloff YG, Carre L, Lavigne AC, Davidson I. The human transcription factor IID subunit human TATA-binding protein-associated factor 28 interacts in a ligand-reversible manner with the vitamin D(3) and thyroid hormone receptors. J Biol Chem 2000;275(14):10064–71.
[41] Kurihara N, Reddy SV, Araki N, et al. Role of TAFII-17, a VDR binding protein, in the increased osteoclast formation in Paget's Disease. J Bone Miner Res 2004;19 (7):1154–64.
[42] Teramachi J, Hiruma Y, Ishizuka S, et al. Role of ATF7-TAF12 interactions in the vitamin D response hypersensitivity of osteoclast precursors in Paget's disease. J Bone Miner Res 2013;28(6):1489–500.
[43] Xing L, Xiu Y, Boyce BF. Osteoclast fusion and regulation by RANKL-dependent and independent factors. World J Orthop 2012;3(12):212–22.
[44] Sarmasik A, Hiruma Y, Okumura S, et al. Measles virus nucleoprotein (MVNP) enhances NFATc1 activation during osteoclastogenesis in Paget's Disease. J Bone Miner Res 2007;22(Suppl 1):S221.
[45] Shanmugarajan S, Youssef RF, Pati P, Ries WL, Rao DS, Reddy SV. Osteoclast inhibitory peptide-1 (OIP-1) inhibits measles virus nucleocapsid protein stimulated osteoclast formation/activity. J Cell Biochem 2008;104(4):1500–8.
[46] Roodman GD, Kurihara N, Ohsaki Y, et al. Interleukin 6. A potential autocrine/ paracrine factor in Paget's disease of bone. J Clin Invest 1992;89(1):46–52.
[47] Menaa C, Reddy SV, Kurihara N, et al. Enhanced RANK ligand expression and responsivity of bone marrow cells in Paget's disease of bone. J Clin Invest 2000;105 (12):1833–8.
[48] Teramachi J, Zhou H, Subler MA, et al. Increased IL-6 expression in osteoclasts is necessary but not sufficient for the development of Paget's disease of bone. J Bone Miner Res 2014;29(6):1456–65.
[49] Keller ET, Wanagat J, Ershler WB. Molecular and cellular biology of interleukin-6 and its receptor. Front Biosci 1996;1:d340–57.
[50] Brunet A, Bonni A, Zigmond MJ, et al. Akt promotes cell survival by phosphorylating and inhibiting a Forkhead transcription factor. Cell 1999;96(6):857–68.
[51] Luron L, Saliba D, Blazek K, Lanfrancotti A, Udalova IA. FOXO3 as a new IKK-epsilon-controlled check-point of regulation of IFN-beta expression. Eur J Immunol 2012;42(4):1030–7.
[52] Yang JY, Zong CS, Xia W, et al. ERK promotes tumorigenesis by inhibiting FOXO3a via MDM2-mediated degradation. Nat Cell Biol 2008;10(2):138–48.
[53] Zajac AJ, Phillips PE. Paget's disease of bone: clinical features and treatment. Clin Exp Rheumatol 1985;3(1):75–88.
[54] Matsuo K, Otaki N. Bone cell interactions through Eph/ephrin: bone modeling, remodeling and associated diseases. Cell Adh Migr 2012;6(2):148–56.
[55] Kurihara N, Teramachi J, Kitagawa Y, Windle JJ, Roodman GD. IGF1 contributes to the increased bone formation induced by measles virus nucleocapsid protein expressed by osteoclasts in Paget's bone disease. J Bone Miner Res 2013;28(Suppl 1): S73.
[56] Teramachi J, Inagaki Y, Mohammad K, et al. Measles virus nucelocapsid protein increases IL-6 and OGF1 in osteoclasts to enhance osteoblast differentiation in Paget's disease. J Bone Miner Res 2015;30(Suppl 1):S380.
[57] Zhang M, Xuan S, Bouxsein ML, et al. Osteoblast-specific knockout of the insulin-like growth factor (IGF) receptor gene reveals an essential role of IGF signaling in bone matrix mineralization. J Biol Chem 2002;277(46):44005–12.

[58] Sundaram K, Senn J, Yuvaraj S, Rao DS, Reddy SV. FGF-2 stimulation of RANK ligand expression in Paget's disease of bone. Mol Endocrinol 2009;23(9):1445–54.
[59] Zhang X, Sobue T, Hurley MM. FGF-2 increases colony formation, PTH receptor, and IGF-1 mRNA in mouse marrow stromal cells. Biochem Biophys Res Commun 2002;290(1):526–31.
[60] Sundaram K, Rao DS, Ries WL, Reddy SV. CXCL5 stimulation of RANK ligand expression in Paget's disease of bone. Lab Invest 2013;93(4):472–9.

CHAPTER 5

Mutant SQSTM1/p62 Signaling in Paget's Disease of Bone

Sarah L. Rea[1,2] and Rob Layfield[3]
[1]Harry Perkins Institute of Medical Research, University of Western Australia, Nedlands, WA, Australia
[2]Department of Endocrinology and Diabetes, Sir Charles Gairdner Hospital, Nedlands, WA, Australia
[3]School of Life Sciences, University of Nottingham, Nottingham, United Kingdom

INTRODUCTION

Paget's disease of bone (PDB) is characterized by focal lesions of excessive bone turnover, initiated by hyperactive osteoclasts and compensated for by changes in osteoblast activity [1]. The primary defect in PDB appears to reside in bone-resorbing osteoclasts, although inherent abnormalities (eg, dysregulated gene expression) have been reported in bone-forming osteoblasts. Pagetic osteoclasts have increased nuclei number per cell compared with normal osteoclasts, increased resorptive capacity, and cell numbers are increased within lesions. Mutations in the *SQSTM1/p62* gene are common in patients with hereditary and sporadic PDB [2], and can also occur de novo (P392L) within lesions [3]. However, the exact mechanisms by which these mutations contribute to disease pathogenesis are not well defined. It is clear that the SQSTM1/p62 protein has important regulatory roles in several cellular signaling pathways that have relevance to osteoclast differentiation, activity, or survival, including nuclear factor kappa B (NFκB) signaling, the oxidative-stress induced Keap1/Nrf2 pathway, and apoptosis [4]. In addition, SQSTM1/p62 regulates protein turnover. These functions of SQSTM1/p62 are interregulated, with defects in one signaling pathway likely to cause changes in another. We outline the current understanding of the impact of mutant SQSTM1/p62 on these pathways with respect to the pathophysiology of PDB.

RANKL-INDUCED NFκB SIGNALING AND OSTEOCLASTOGENESIS

Although bones from 6- to 8-week-old *SQSTM1/p62* knockout mice appear histologically normal, bone resorption in response to parathyroid

S.V. Reddy (Ed): Advances in Pathobiology and Management of Paget's Disease of Bone.
DOI: http://dx.doi.org/10.1016/B978-0-12-805083-5.00005-1

hormone-related protein (PTHrP) challenge is impaired, indicating a role for SQSTM1/p62 in stress-induced bone resorption [5]. PTHrP induces osteoclast formation indirectly by stimulating osteoblastic Receptor activator of NFκB ligand (RANKL) expression, yet the RANKL levels produced were similar between knockout and wild-type mice, consistent with a role for SQSTM1/p62 downstream of RANKL. It is noteworthy that stromal cells from transgenic mice expressing the mouse equivalent of the most common PDB-associated P392L mutation of SQSTM1/p62 (P394L in mice) produce increased RANKL, promoting enhanced osteoclastogenesis [6].

Osteoclasts form via fusion of precursor monocytes into a multinucleated, terminally differentiated cell; this occurs following the binding of RANKL, expressed by osteoblasts, to its cognate receptor RANK expressed at the cell surface on the preosteoclast (Fig. 5.1). Osteoclast precursor cells isolated from PDB patients are hyperresponsive to RANKL, as well as 1,25$(OH)_2$ vitamin D_3 [7,8], which may partially account for the increased osteoclast number and activity that occur in lesions. In conjunction with macrophage-colony stimulating factor (M-CSF), RANKL induces osteoclast differentiation via TNF receptor associated factor-6 (TRAF6)-dependent activation of mitogen activated protein kinase (MAPK) pathways (p38, JNK, ERK) and the serine/threonine kinase Akt. This leads to osteoclast-specific gene expression via the activation of transcription factors, including NFκB, activator protein 1 (AP-1; a dimer comprised of variously combined Jun, Fos or ATF family members), and nuclear factor of activated T-cells (NFATc1) (Fig. 5.1). TRAF6 is a critical adaptor protein for RANK in osteoclasts; mice lacking TRAF6, NFκB, or c-Fos (AP-1) develop osteopetrosis due to defects in osteoclast formation and/or bone resorption [9].

TRAF6 is an E3 ubiquitin ligase that is activated via autoubiquitination in an SQSTM1/p62-dependent manner, as TRAF6 from the brains of *SQSTM1/p62* knockout mice is not ubiquitin-modified [10]. In response to RANKL stimulation of precursor osteoclasts, SQSTM1/p62 forms a ternary complex with TRAF6 and an atypical protein kinase C isoform (PKCζ/λ) leading to activation of the inhibitor of κB (IκB) kinase (IKK), subsequent phosphorylation and degradation of IκB and release of NFκB to the nucleus (Fig. 5.2) [5]. The role of SQSTM1/p62 in RANKL-induced NFκB signaling may be biphasic. Bone marrow-derived monocytes (BMDMs) do not require SQSTM1/p62 for NFκB activation by RANKL in the early stages (30 minutes posttreatment), yet activation was

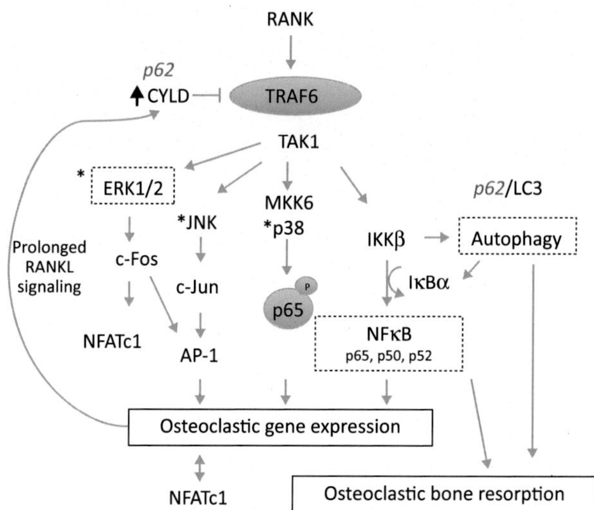

Figure 5.1 RANK signaling in osteoclasts. Osteoclast differentiation requires activation of several essential transcription factors including NFκB, AP-1 and NFATc1 by upstream kinases. An essential adaptor protein for RANK is TRAF6, an E3-ubiquitin ligase that is activated by auto-ubiquitination. TRAF6 activates TAK1 kinase, which in turn is required for activation of the MAPKs (*ERK, p38 and JNK). The MAPKs are also activated by RANKL-induced ROS; this may be downstream of TAK1. TAK1-dependent phosphorylation of the NFκB subunit p65/RelA is now known to be essential for osteoclast formation, yet TAK1 also phosphorylates IKKβ. In addition to roles in osteoclastogenesis, NFκB and ERK1/2 are important for cell survival. Furthermore, NFκB and autophagy are important for osteoclastic bone resorption (indicated by dashed boxes). Downregulation of osteoclastogenesis occurs via SQSTM1/p62 (indicated p62)-dependent bridging of CYLD (a deubiquitinating enzyme) with TRAF6, this leads to TRAF6 de-activation, inhibited NFκB activity, and attenuation of osteoclastogenesis.

markedly reduced in SQSTM1/p62-deficient BMDMs following 1–2 days RANKL treatment [5]. This study appears at odds with several reports that SQSTM1/p62 may act as a negative regulator of NFκB signaling, since in vitro overexpression leads to inhibition of NFκB activity compared with empty vector controls [2,11–13]. Negative regulation of NFκB by SQSTM1/p62 also attenuates osteoblast differentiation [14].

DEFECTIVE NFκB SIGNALING ASSOCIATED WITH MUTANT SQSTM1/p62

The regulation of the NFκB pathway in osteoclasts by wild-type SQSTM1/p62 is facilitated at least in part via a scaffolding function that

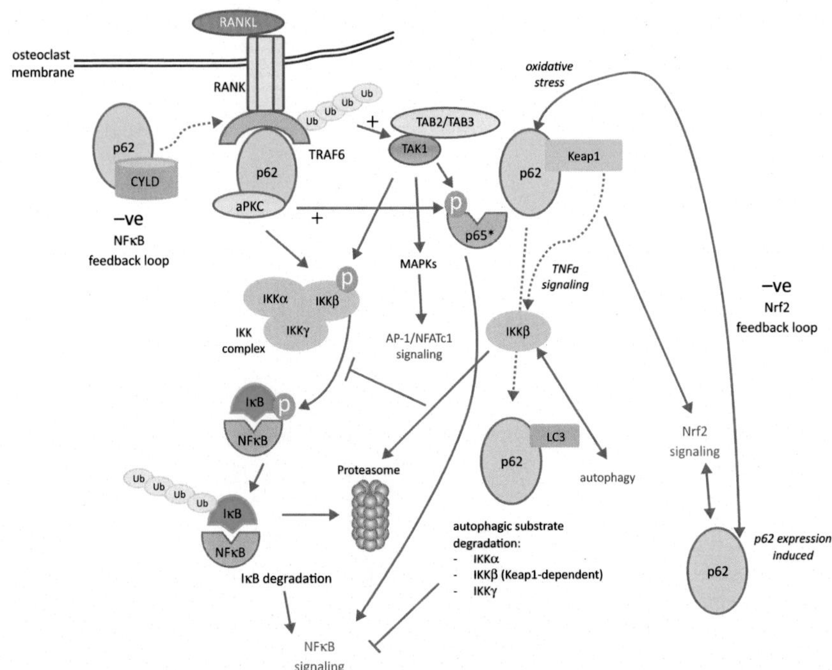

Figure 5.2 Regulation of osteoclast signaling by SQSTM1/p62. Osteoclast signaling responses to RANKL stimulation are relayed downstream by effector molecules. SQSTM1/p62 (indicated p62) is implicated in TRAF6 activation via ubiquitination. Active TRAF6 is required for TAK1 regulation of NFκB, AP-1, and NFATc1, and also forms a ternary complex with SQSTM1/p62 and aPKC. As osteoclastogenesis progresses, CYLD expression is increased and SQSTM1/p62 facilitates a negative feedback inhibition by acting as a bridge between CYLD and TRAF6. PDB-associated mutant proteins (UBA-truncated and P392L) do not interact with CYLD and are associated with increased NFκB signaling. Autophagy also regulates IKK subunits and in TNFα signaling specifically, is mediated by Keap1. SQSTM1/p62 is upregulated during oxidative stress and outcompetes Nrf2 for Keap1 binding, leading to increased Nrf2 activity. RANKL induces ROS production, which may also affect Nrf2 signaling in osteoclasts.

physically links ubiquitinated TRAF6 with the deubiquitinating enzyme cylindromatosis (CYLD). This leads to decreased levels of ubiquitinated TRAF6, decreased NFκB activity, and attenuated osteoclastogenesis [15], whereas the expression of PDB-associated mutant SQSTM1/p62 proteins in vitro increases osteoclastogenesis and bone resorption and this appears to be mediated by increased NFκB signaling [12,13,16]. Several groups have now reported that PDB-associated missense and truncating mutations affecting the ubiquitin-associated (UBA) domain of SQSTM1/p62, and at least two non-UBA domain mutations, are associated with increased NFκB activity relative to wild-type, but not always to levels above the empty vector control [11–13]. Thus, mutant SQSTM1/p62 proteins have a diminished capacity for inhibiting NFκB signaling. In some cases, the underlying mechanism was shown to be due to a defect in the deubiquitination of TRAF6 by CYLD [15] (Fig. 5.2). Importantly, this regulation requires the ubiquitin-binding ability of the UBA domain, as UBA-deficient SQSTM1/p62, and ubiquitin-binding impaired (P392L) proteins fail to interact with CYLD. However, a non-UBA domain PDB mutant protein (A381V) retains interaction with CYLD [17] despite a previous study showing that this mutant increases activation of NFκB [11]. Together, these studies highlight the possibility that for different PDB mutant SQSTM1/p62 proteins distinct mechanisms may be involved in disease induction and/or progression.

It has been suggested that the inhibition of NFκB signaling by SQSTM1/p62 may be due to altered proteasomal degradation of IκB [18]. The authors found that relative to wild-type and control cells, osteoclasts expressing the P392L mutant SQSTM1/p62 protein had increased levels of IκB, due to decreased interaction and shuttling to the proteasome, yet paradoxically NFκB was hyperactivated [18]. Indeed a previous report showed that osteoclasts overexpressing P392L mutant SQSTM1/p62 are constitutively active, with increased levels of activated PKCζ/λ and NFκB activity prior to RANKL stimuli [16]. One study suggests that increased NFκB activity associated with mutant P392L SQSTM1/p62 protein may partially be imparted by preferential activation of an alternative NFκB pathway involving PKCζ-induced phosphorylation of the NFκB subunit p65 (RelA) at S536 [18].

Alternatively, signaling regulation may be intimately linked with the ability of SQSTM1/p62 to engage with ubiquitin or ubiquitinated partner proteins. The majority of PDB mutations reported to date affect the UBA domain of SQSTM1/p62. As such, the effect of various mutations on the ability of SQSTM1/p62 to bind ubiquitin (which appears related to its ability to regulate TRAF6) has been studied. Missense and truncating mutations affecting the UBA domain lead to markedly reduced or abolished ubiquitin-binding [19], whereas non-UBA mutant proteins (ie, P364S and A381V) retain the ability to bind ubiquitin while still eliciting increased activation of NFκB [2,11]. This indicates that reduced ubiquitin-binding per se may not be the mechanism underlying increased NFκB signaling in osteoclasts. These studies do not rule out the possibility that interaction between SQSTM1/p62 and specific ubiquitinated substrate proteins may be affected by mutations and lead to increased signaling. Our recent study showed that mutations within the UBA domain exert distinct effects on protein structure and function, although both ultimately decrease ubiquitin-binding and hyperactivate NFκB [20].

SQSTM1/P62-MEDIATED RANKL-INDUCED AP-1, NFAT, AND ERK SIGNALING

Hyperactivation of additional RANKL-induced signaling pathways, namely AP-1, NFATc1, and ERK, has been reported in PDB with *SQSTM1/p62* mutations. Two studies have reported increased activity of AP-1 associated with P392L mutant SQSTM1/p62 protein expression [4,17]. In addition, the non-UBA domain P364S mutation and a UBA-deficient mutant protein (K378X) also elicited increased AP-1 activity [4]. In agreement with this, an earlier study showed increased RANKL-induced NFATc1 and ERK in $RAW_{264.7}$ cells stably expressing UBA-deficient SQSTM1/p62 [12]. NFATc1 and ERK pathways are involved in osteoclastogenesis, with NFATc1 regarded as the master regulator of osteoclastogenesis downstream of NFκB and AP-1; ERK pathways also induce osteoclast formation. Altogether, these studies suggest that SQSTM1/p62 is important for the regulation of osteoclasts via multiple RANKL-induced pathways, and that the mechanisms underlying mutation pathogenesis is to increase the osteoclastic potential of precursor cells [6].

SQSTM1/P62-MEDIATED REGULATION OF Keap1/Nrf2 SIGNALING

Long-lived reactive oxygen species (ROS) are produced in response to RANKL stimulation and activate p38, JNK, and ERK MAPKs. In addition to crucial roles in osteoclast formation and regulation of bone resorption, bone homeostasis is also maintained by ROS through the inhibition of osteoblasts [21]. Although the role of the Nrf2 transcription factor in osteoclasts is not well defined, inhibitors of RANKL-mediated ROS generation lead to decreased osteoclast formation via the upregulation of Nrf2 dependent antioxidant gene transcription. In nonstimulated cells, Keap1 is a negative regulator of Nrf2 that mediates the constitutive degradation of the transcription factor by the 26S proteasome. In response to oxidative or electrophilic stressors Keap1 is inactivated and this leads to stabilization of Nrf2 and subsequent expression of various detoxifying and antioxidant genes [22].

Recently SQSTM1/p62 was identified as a positive feedback modulator of Nrf2. SQSTM1/p62 expression is induced in response to oxidative stress and leads to increased levels of Nrf2. SQSTM1/p62 interacts with Keap1 via its Keap1-interacting region (KIR) which spans amino acid residues 347–352. The binding site on Keap1 for SQSTM1/p62 overlaps with one of two Nrf2 binding sites, thus Nrf2 is liberated due to the competitive binding of SQSTM1/p62 to Keap1 [22]. We recently characterized a PDB-associated non-UBA domain SQSTM1/p62 mutation (S349T) and found that unlike other mutations it had no effect on ubiquitin-binding or basal NFκB signaling. However, the mutation affects a residue within the KIR and decreases SQSTM1/p62 interaction with Keap1, leading to reduced induction of Nrf2 activity [23]. The mechanisms through which decreased activation of Nrf2 might contribute to PDB are not yet known, it is likely that altered basal Nrf2 activity would have effects on osteoclast and osteoblast differentiation. This study provides further evidence that diverse disease mechanisms may be involved in PDB with *SQSTM1/p62* mutations.

SQSTM1/p62-MEDIATED APOPTOSIS

SQSTM1/p62 controls the aggregation of proteins that are destined for degradation by autophagy as a mechanism of cell protection (see below). However, it also facilitates apoptotic cell death, a process central to determining the lifespan of osteoclasts. Regulation of apoptosis can be via an autophagy membrane-dependent mechanism; specifically SQSTM1/p62 regulates caspase-8, a critical initiator of the extrinsic apoptosis pathway [24]. Caspase-8 is recruited to the death-inducing signaling complex (DISC) following stimulation of cell-surface death receptors (DR). Stimulation of DR4 or DR5 with the proapoptotic ligand TNF-related apoptosis inducing ligand (TRAIL) leads to proximity-induced dimerization of caspase-8. This dimerization supports an initial stimulation of the protease, but for cellular commitment to apoptosis aggregation of caspase-8 is required, which is facilitated by SQSTM1/p62. Knockdown of SQSTM1/p62 decreases active caspase-8 and attenuates TRAIL-induced apoptosis highlighting its critical role in facilitating apoptosis [24]. Young et al. show that the autophagosomal membrane provides a platform for an intracellular DISC [25] that has previously been reported as essential for initiation of the caspase-8/-3 cascade [24]. These studies together suggest a model whereby the association of SQSTM1/p62 with the autophagy protein LC3-II links self-associated caspase-8 with the autophagosomal membrane, where the caspase-8 can then self-activate via oligomerization [25]. Recently it has been shown that SQSTM1/p62 is itself cleaved by caspase-8 in an RIPK-dependent manner. This cleavage prevents SQSTM1/p62-LC3 complex formation, suggesting that autophagy may be downregulated during necroptosis. However, the significance of these findings, particularly with regard to pathological situations, is not yet known [26].

Importantly abnormal apoptosis has been detected in osteoclasts derived from peripheral blood mononuclear cells (PBMCs) of PDB patients. Proapoptotic genes were downregulated in PDB-derived osteoclasts compared with healthy controls, specifically the *CASP3* (Caspase-3) and *TNFRSF10A* (TRAIL-R1) genes [27]. However, no significant difference was observed when comparing expression levels of these genes in osteoclasts from PDB patients with the SQSTM1/p62 P392L mutation and those without [27]. Further, increased expression of the apoptosis inhibitor *Bcl2* has been reported in Pagetic osteoclasts [28]. A study of human PBMC-derived osteoclasts determined the percentage of cells undergoing apoptosis in response to (1) withdrawal of the survival cytokines RANKL and M-CSF, or (2) TRAIL stimulation: apoptosis was decreased compared to healthy donor (HD) controls in PDB-derived osteoclasts (with or without *SQSTM1/p62* mutation) and was also decreased in HD osteoclasts carrying the P392L mutation [16]. These studies strongly implicate impaired apoptosis of osteoclasts in PDB pathophysiology. However, the presence of the P392L mutation of SQSTM1/p62 in cells from PDB-patients did not lead to any further reduction in apoptosis, as apoptosis of PDB-derived osteoclasts lacking the mutation was similarly reduced. While it is possible that SQSTM1/p62 mutations have a direct effect on apoptosis pathways, perhaps via dysfunctional autophagy (see below), the increase in NFκB survival signaling may also contribute to increased protection in times of cellular stress that normally lead to apoptosis, such as the withdrawal of RANKL and M-CSF.

SQSTM1/p62-MEDIATED AUTOPHAGY

Macroautophagy (hereafter, autophagy) is a degradative process used to protect cells against insults that may be caused due to long-lived proteins, protein aggregates, and damaged or excessive organelles. Autophagy is induced to help cells survive starvation, however it may also lead to cell death through self-cannibalization or the activation of apoptosis [29]. In the initial step of autophagy a double membrane-bound structure forms surrounding substrates, referred to as an autophagosome. The autophagosome undergoes fusion with a lysosome or an endosome to form an autophagolysosome. Lysosomal enzymes then degrade the sequestered materials. Autophagy was initially thought to be a nonselective process. We now know that SQSTM1/p62 acts as a critical "receptor" which selects specific ubiquitinated substrate proteins for incorporation into autophagolysosomes, a process that involves protein aggregation and the physical interaction of SQSTM1/p62 with the autophagy protein LC3 [30]. This human homolog of the autophagy protein Atg8 can be cytosolic (LC3-I) or may be lipidated and membrane-bound (LC3-II). The latter form promotes autophagosome fusion with lysosomes; as such LC3-II is often identified as a late marker of autophagy.

Recently, autophagy was found to play noncanonical roles in the regulation of osteoclasts [31]. LC3 was shown to localize to the ruffled border of osteoclasts. Additionally, the critical autophagy proteins (Atg5, Atg7, and Atg4B) were reported to be important regulators of bone resorption [32]. Notably, increased levels of LC3-II accumulate in osteoclasts from SQSTM1/p62^{P394L} mice treated with the lysosomal inhibitor Bafilomycin compared with wild-type littermates, consistent with dysregulation of autophagy and enhanced autophagosome formation [33]. We have observed dysfunctional autophagy associated with mutant SQSTM1/p62 protein expression in cell models (unpublished data) as have another group [34]. Therefore it seems likely that disturbed autophagy may be involved in disease pathogenesis in PDB with *SQSTM1/p62* mutations. Recently, mutations in SQSTM1/p62 have also been reported in patients with amyotrophic lateral sclerosis (ALS) and frontotemporal dementia, including some mutations that are associated with PDB [35]. A zebrafish SQSTM1/p62 knockdown model of ALS showed that the locomotor effects could be rescued by the autophagy activator rapamycin or reintroduction of human SQSTM1/p62, but not by introduction of disease-associated SQSTM1/p62 UBA domain mutants. This indicates that a defective UBA domain is leading to disturbed autophagy in this model; accordingly, in the SQSTM1/p62 knockdown zebrafish increased levels of the autophagy inhibitor mTOR were reported [36].

Parkin-PINK1 mediated mitophagy, the specific autophagy of mitochondria, is impaired by mutations in VCP, which cause the multisystem proteinopathy Inclusion body myopathy with PDB and frontotemporal dementia [37]. Mitochondrial biogenesis is linked to RANKL-induced OCL differentiation and function. Recently, the phosphorylation of S403 within the UBA domain of SQSTM1/p62 by TANK-binding kinase 1 was shown to be required for the autophagosomal engulfment of parkin-recruited mitochondria [38]. Given the vast majority of PDB-associated mutations affect the UBA domain of SQSTM1/p62, it will be interesting to investigate the affect of such mutations on mitophagy in osteoclasts.

The charged multivesicular body protein 5 (CHMP5) is a component of the endosomal sorting complex required for transport (ESCRT) machinery, which has roles in autophagy, and also downregulation of signaling through receptor degradation. Conditional deletion of the *CHMP5* gene (in osteoclasts) leads to a high bone turnover phenotype in mice that significantly resembles PDB [39]. Notably polymorphisms in several other autophagy genes have recently been associated with PDB in a Spanish cohort [40]. These studies further implicate autophagy as key to PDB pathogenesis.

SQSTM1/p62 AS A SIGNALING HUB ORCHESTRATING THE INTERPLAY BETWEEN NFκB, Keap1 AND AUTOPHAGY

The essential mediator of NFκB activation, IKK, was recently identified as fundamental for autophagy induction, with activation of IKK shown to be both sufficient and required for optimal autophagy induction in response to various stimuli [41]. Furthermore, TNFα-induced NFκB activation requires the essential autophagy proteins Atg5 and Atg7 and autophagy modulators Beclin 1 and VPS34, as knockdown of these proteins results in inhibition of NFκB [42]. Additional links between NFκB and autophagy are found in the autophagy mediator Beclin 1 and TAK1-binding proteins (TAB) 2 and 3 [43], which are upstream activators of the TAK1-IKK signaling cascade in RANKL, TNFα, and IL-1 signaling. In "resting" cells, TAB2 and TAB3 are bound to Beclin 1. In response to autophagy inducers, the TAB proteins dissociate from Beclin 1 and bind to TAK1. This molecular switch in the cell turns the inhibition of autophagy off, as TAK1 activation of IKKβ leads to induction of autophagy [43]. These studies highlight that the NFκB and autophagy pathways have significant commonality. Importantly, RANKL-induced Beclin 1 expression leads to ROS induction of JNK/p38 and downstream NFATc1 activation, inhibition of Beclin 1 inhibits OCL formation [44]. Further, the Nrf2 regulatory protein and binding partner

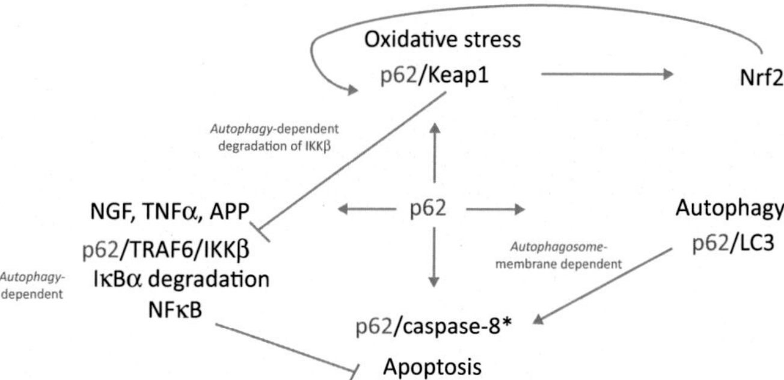

Figure 5.3 SQSTM1/p62 as a signaling hub. Survival signaling through NFκB (induced by RANKL, TNFα, and IL-1 in osteoclasts) is regulated in part via complex formation of SQSTM1/p62 (indicated p62) with aPKC, which leads to the activation of IKKβ and subsequent phosphorylation and autophagy (SQSTM1/p62-dependent) degradation of IκB. TNFα signaling leads to IKKβ degradation *via* autophagy in a Keap1-dependent manner, while IKKβ itself induces autophagy in an NFκB-independent manner linking NFκB with both oxidative signaling and autophagy. In addition to linkage with autophagy, NFκB also leads to inhibition of apoptosis. TRAIL-induced apoptosis requires SQSTM1/p62-dependent aggregation of caspase-8, and SQSTM1/p62 interaction with the autophagosomal membrane.

of SQSTM1/p62, Keap1, downregulates TNFα-induced activation of NFκB by facilitating the autophagic degradation of IKKβ [45], thus linking not only NFκB and autophagy, but also the oxidative stress pathways via SQSTM1/p62. For this reason, SQSTM1/p62 is referred to as a "signaling hub" (Fig. 5.3). Importantly, various stressors including starvation, infection, proteasome inhibition, NFκB activation and Nrf2 activation upregulate SQSTM1/p62.

SQSTM1/p62 is primarily localized in cytoplasmic aggregates or "speckles." It has been suggested that these speckles are the location of "signal-organizing centers" where SQSTM1/p62 may favor the formation of particular signaling complexes with different molecules in response to a variety of cell stimuli and thereby regulate the decisions between cell survival and apoptosis. However, the specific temporal and spatial conditions modulating these decisions are yet to be elucidated [46].

With relation to PDB, it is clear that the expression of mutant SQSTM1/p62 proteins lead to enhanced signaling, which favor osteoclastogenesis (Table 5.1). Studies to date show that most, but not all of these mutations disrupt ubiquitin-binding by SQSTM1/p62 and most, but not all lead to increased NFκB signaling. In some cases this may be due to either decreased negative regulation via an inability to bind CYLD and/

Table 5.1 Effects of *SQSTM1* mutations associated with PDB on cellular signaling pathways

Pathway	Significance	Effect of mutations	Mechanism(s)
NFκB signaling	Promotes osteoclastogenesis, osteoclast survival and activity	Diminished capacity for inhibiting RANK-NFκB signaling	• Impaired CYLD-mediated deubiquitination of TRAF6?? • Preferential activation (PKCζ-mediated) of the NFκB subunit p65 (RelA)??
AP-1 signaling	Promotes osteoclastogenesis	Activation of AP-1	Unknown[a]
NFATc1 signaling	Promotes osteoclastogenesis	Activation of NFATc1	Unknown[a]
ERK signaling	Promotes osteoclastogenesis and osteoclast survival	Activation of ERK	Unknown[a]
Keap1/Nrf2 signaling	Regulates expression of various detoxifying and antioxidant genes	Reduced induction of Nrf2 activity[b]	Impaired SQSTM1/p62 binding to Keap1[b]
Autophagy	Removal of osteoclasts after bone resorption. Autophagy proteins have roles in delivery of Cathepsin K to the ruffled border for resorption	Dysregulation of autophagy—enhanced autophagy markers (LC3-II)	Unknown

[a]May result from upstream changes in RANK-NFκB signaling pathway.
[b]Only for S349T mutation.

or a constitutive activation of PKCζ. To date only one PDB mutant SQSTM1/p62 has been reported to inhibit Nrf2 activity, leading to a decrease in basal antioxidant gene expression, which could affect bone cell differentiation. Together these studies suggest that distinct mechanisms may be involved in PDB pathogenesis. However, our unpublished work, and that of others suggests that SQSTM1/p62 mutant proteins are consistently defective in their ability to regulate autophagy. This is also supported by an increase in autophagic flux noted in SQSTM1/p62^{P394L} mice [33]. Given the vast overlap between the signaling pathways involving SQSTM1/p62, it is likely that PDB mutant proteins with impaired ability to mediate autophagy would lead to downstream effects on multiple signaling pathways (and vice versa). Intriguingly, the severity of Pagetic phenotype in offspring that have inherited SQSTM1/p62 mutations is attenuated compared to that of their parent and disease onset is also delayed. This strongly suggests that although *SQSTM1* gene mutations are important, gene–environment interactions are also likely to impact disease progression [47].

REFERENCES

[1] Naot D, Bava U, Matthews B, Callon KE, Gamble GD, Black M, et al. Differential gene expression in cultured osteoblasts and bone marrow stromal cells from patients with Paget's disease of bone. J Bone Miner Res 2007;22(2):298–309.

[2] Rea SL, Walsh JP, Ward L, Magno AL, Ward BK, Shaw B, et al. Sequestosome 1 mutations in Paget's disease of bone in Australia: prevalence, genotype/phenotype correlation, and a novel non-UBA domain mutation (P364S) associated with increased NF-kappaB signaling without loss of ubiquitin binding. J Bone Miner Res 2009;24(7):1216–23.

[3] Guay-Bélanger S, Picard S, Gagnon E, Morissette J, Siris ES, Orcel P, et al. Detection of SQSTM1/P392L post-zygotic mutations in Paget's disease of bone. Hum Genet 2015;134(1):53–65.

[4] Rea SL, Walsh JP, Layfield R, Ratajczak T, Xu J. New insights into the role of sequestosome 1/p62 mutant proteins in the pathogenesis of Paget's disease of bone. Endocrine Rev 2013;34(4):501–24.

[5] Duran A, Serrano M, Leitges M, Flores JM, Picard S, Brown JP, et al. The atypical PKC-interacting protein p62 is an important mediator of RANK-activated osteoclastogenesis. Dev Cell 2004;6(2):303–9.

[6] Hiruma Y, Kurihara N, Subler MA, Zhou H, Boykin CS, Zhang H, et al. A SQSTM1/p62 mutation linked to Paget's disease increases the osteoclastogenic potential of the bone microenvironment. Hum Mol Genet 2008;17(23):3708–19.

[7] Neale SD, Smith R, Wass JA, Athanasou NA. Osteoclast differentiation from circulating mononuclear precursors in Paget's disease is hypersensitive to 1,25-dihydroxyvitamin D(3) and RANKL. Bone 2000;27(3):409–16.

[8] Roodman GD. Insights into the pathogenesis of Paget's disease. Ann N Y Acad Sci 2010;1192:176–80.

[9] Tolar J, Teitelbaum SL, Orchard PJ. Osteopetrosis. N Engl J Med 2004;351 (27):2839–49.
[10] Wooten MW, Geetha T, Seibenhener ML, Babu JR, Diaz-Meco MT, Moscat J. The p62 scaffold regulates nerve growth factor-induced NF-kappaB activation by influencing TRAF6 polyubiquitination. J Biol Chem 2005;280(42):35625–9.
[11] Najat D, Garner T, Hagen T, Shaw B, Sheppard PW, Falchetti A, et al. Characterization of a non-UBA domain missense mutation of sequestosome 1 (SQSTM1) in Paget's disease of bone. J Bone Miner Res 2009;24(4):632–42.
[12] Yip KH, Feng H, Pavlos NJ, Zheng MH, Xu J. p62 ubiquitin binding-associated domain mediated the receptor activator of nuclear factor-kappaB ligand-induced osteoclast formation: a new insight into the pathogenesis of Paget's disease of bone. Am J Pathol 2006;169(2):503–14.
[13] Rea SL, Walsh JP, Ward L, Yip K, Ward BK, Kent GN, et al. A novel mutation (K378X) in the sequestosome 1 gene associated with increased NF-kappaB signaling and Paget's disease of bone with a severe phenotype. J Bone Miner Res 2006;21 (7):1136–45.
[14] Chang KH, Sengupta A, Nayak RC, Duran A, Lee SJ, Pratt RG, et al. p62 is required for stem cell/progenitor retention through inhibition of IKK/NF-κB/Ccl4 signaling at the bone marrow macrophage-osteoblast niche. Cell Rep 2014;9 (6):2084–97.
[15] Jin W, Chang M, Paul EM, Babu G, Lee AJ, Reiley W, et al. Deubiquitinating enzyme CYLD negatively regulates RANK signaling and osteoclastogenesis in mice. J Clin Invest 2008;118(5):1858–66.
[16] Chamoux E, Couture J, Bisson M, Morissette J, Brown JP, Roux S. The p62 P392L mutation linked to Paget's disease induces activation of human osteoclasts. Mol Endocrinol 2009;23(10):1668–80.
[17] Sundaram K, Shanmugarajan S, Rao DS, Reddy SV. Mutant p62P392L stimulation of osteoclast differentiation in Paget's disease of bone. Endocrinology 2011;152(11):4180–9.
[18] Chamoux E, McManus S, Laberge G, Bisson M, Roux S. Involvement of kinase PKC-zeta in the p62/p62(P392L)-driven activation of NF-kappaB in human osteoclasts. Biochim Biophys Acta 2013;1832(3):475–84.
[19] Cavey JR, Ralston SH, Hocking LJ, Sheppard PW, Ciani B, Searle MS, et al. Loss of ubiquitin-binding associated with Paget's disease of bone p62 (SQSTM1) mutations. J Bone Miner Res 2005;20(4):619–24.
[20] Goode A, Long JE, Shaw B, Ralston SH, Visconti MR, Gianfrancesco F, et al. Paget disease of bone-associated UBA domain mutations of SQSTM1 exerts distinct effects on protein structure and function. Biochim Biophys Acta 2014.
[21] Kousteni S. FoxOs: unifying links between oxidative stress and skeletal homeostasis. Curr Osteoporos Rep 2011;9(2):60–6.
[22] Komatsu M, Kurokawa H, Waguri S, Taguchi K, Kobayashi A, Ichimura Y, et al. The selective autophagy substrate p62 activates the stress responsive transcription factor Nrf2 through inactivation of Keap1. Nat Cell Biol 2010;12(3):213–23.
[23] Wright T, Rea SL, Goode A, Bennett AJ, Ratajczak T, Long JE, et al. The S349T mutation of SQSTM1 links Keap1/Nrf2 signalling to Paget's disease of bone. Bone 2013;52(2):699–706.
[24] Jin Z, Li Y, Pitti R, Lawrence D, Pham VC, Lill JR, et al. Cullin3-based polyubiquitination and p62-dependent aggregation of caspase-8 mediate extrinsic apoptosis signaling. Cell 2009;137(4):721–35.
[25] Young M, Takahashi Y, Khan O, Park S, Hori T, Yun J, et al. Autophagosomal membrane serves as a platform for an intracellular death-inducing signaling complex

(iDISC)-mediated caspase-8 activation and apoptosis. J Biol Chem 2012;287 (15):12455–68.

[26] Matsuzawa Y, Oshima S, Nibe Y, Kobayashi M, Maeyashiki C, Nemoto Y, et al. RIPK3 regulates p62-LC3 complex formation via the caspase-8-dependent cleavage of p62. Biochem Biophys Res Commun 2015;456(1):298–304.

[27] Michou L, Chamoux E, Couture J, Morissette J, Brown JP, Roux S. Gene expression profile in osteoclasts from patients with Paget's disease of bone. Bone 2010;46 (3):598–603.

[28] Brandwood CP, Hoyland JA, Hillarby MC, Berry JL, Davies M, Selby PL, et al. Apoptotic gene expression in Paget's disease: a possible role for Bcl-2. J Pathol 2003;201(3):504–12.

[29] Levine B, Kroemer G. Autophagy in the pathogenesis of disease. Cell 2008;132 (1):27–42.

[30] Pankiv S, Clausen TH, Lamark T, Brech A, Bruun JA, Outzen H, et al. p62/SQSTM1 binds directly to Atg8/LC3 to facilitate degradation of ubiquitinated protein aggregates by autophagy. J Biol Chem 2007;282(33):24131–45.

[31] Hocking LJ, Whitehouse C, Helfrich MH. Autophagy: a new player in skeletal maintenance? J Bone Miner Res 2012;27(7):1439–47.

[32] DeSelm CJ, Miller BC, Zou W, Beatty WL, van Meel E, Takahata Y, et al. Autophagy proteins regulate the secretory component of osteoclastic bone resorption. Dev Cell 2011;21(5):966–74.

[33] Daroszewska A, van't Hof RJ, Rojas JA, Layfield R, Landao-Basonga E, Rose L, et al. A point mutation in the ubiquitin-associated domain of SQSMT1 is sufficient to cause a Paget's disease-like disorder in mice. Hum Mol Genet 2011;20(14): 2734–44.

[34] Azzam EA, Helfrich MH, Hocking LJ. Paget's disease-causing mutations in Sequestosome-1 impair autophagic degradation. J Bone Miner Res 2011;26 Abstract 1081

[35] Rea SL, Majcher V, Searle MS, Layfield R. SQSTM1 mutations—bridging Paget disease of bone and ALS/FTLD. Exp Cell Res 2014;325(1):27–37.

[36] Lattante S, de Calbiac H, Le Ber I, Brice A, Ciura S, Kabashi E. Sqstm1 knock-down causes a locomotor phenotype ameliorated by rapamycin in a zebrafish model of ALS/FTLD. Hum Mol Genet 2015;24(6):1682–90.

[37] Kim NC, Tresse E, Kolaitis RM, Molliex A, Thomas RE, Alami NH, et al. VCP is essential for mitochondrial quality control by PINK1/Parkin and this function is impaired by VCP mutations. Neuron 2013;78(1):65–80.

[38] Matsumoto G, Shimogori T, Hattori N, Nukina N. TBK1 controls autophagosomal engulfment of polyubiquitinated mitochondria through p62/SQSTM1 phosphorylation. Hum Mol Genet 2015;24(15):4429–42.

[39] Greenblatt MB, Park KH, Oh H, Kim JM, Shin DY, Lee JM, et al. CHMP5 controls bone turnover rates by dampening NF-κB activity in osteoclasts. J Exp Med 2015;212(8):1283–301.

[40] Usategui-Martín R, García-Aparicio J, Corral-Gudino L, Calero-Paniagua I, Del Pino-Montes J, González Sarmiento R. Polymorphisms in autophagy genes are associated with paget disease of bone. Plos One 2015;10(6) e0128984

[41] Criollo A, Senovilla L, Authier H, Maiuri MC, Morselli E, Vitale I, et al. IKK connects autophagy to major stress pathways. Autophagy 2010;6(1):189–91.

[42] Criollo A, Chereau F, Malik SA, Niso-Santano M, Marino G, Galluzzi L, et al. Autophagy is required for the activation of NFkappaB. Cell Cycle 2012;11(1):194–9.

[43] Criollo A, Niso-Santano M, Malik SA, Michaud M, Morselli E, Marino G, et al. Inhibition of autophagy by TAB2 and TAB3. EMBO J 2011;30(24):4908–20.

[44] Chung YH, Jang Y, Choi B, Song DH, Lee EJ, Kim SM, et al. Beclin-1 is required for RANKL-induced osteoclast differentiation. J Cell Physiol 2014;229 (12):1963–71.
[45] Kim JE, You DJ, Lee C, Ahn C, Seong JY, Hwang JI. Suppression of NF-kappaB signaling by KEAP1 regulation of IKKbeta activity through autophagic degradation and inhibition of phosphorylation. Cell Signal 2010;22(11):1645–54.
[46] Nakamura K, Kimple AJ, Siderovski DP, Johnson GL. PB1 domain interaction of p62/sequestosome 1 and MEKK3 regulates NF-kappaB activation. J Biol Chem 2010;285(3):2077–89.
[47] Cundy T, Rutland MD, Naot D, Bolland M. Evolution of Paget's disease of bone in adults inheriting SQSTM1 mutations. Clin Endocrinol (Oxf) 2015;83(3):315–19.

CHAPTER 6

Early Onset Pagetic Disorders: Implications for Late-Onset Paget's Disease of Bone

Julie C. Crockett and Miep H. Helfrich
Musculoskeletal Research Programme, University of Aberdeen, Aberdeen, United Kingdom

INTRODUCTION

Bone remodeling, the balanced activities of bone resorbing osteoclasts and bone forming osteoblasts, occurs throughout life to maintain a healthy skeleton [1]. The key feature of Paget's disease of bone (PDB) is the presence of focal areas of increased bone remodeling. The bone remodeling is driven by osteoclasts, but coupled with increased osteoblast activity, leading to the characteristically high serum alkaline phosphatase levels in patients (see Chapter 1, Clinical Perspectives of Paget's Disease of Bone). In considering the molecular consequences of mutations or other genetic variation associated with development of the skeletal disease, the focus to date has been to elucidate how the genetic change will affect osteoclast development and/or behavior. It is important to remember, however, that the mutations are germline and that all cells in the patient potentially express the mutant protein. More work is still required to assess the contribution of cell types other than osteoclasts to the skeletal phenotype seen in Pagetic disorders. A syndromic condition caused by mutations in the gene for valosin-containing protein (VCP), further discussed below, exemplifies how some mutations can cause disease affecting several tissues. The bone pathology in Pagetic disorders is most clearly demonstrated in osteoclasts and hence the focus of this chapter.

The differentiation, fusion, activity, and survival of osteoclasts is tightly regulated by signaling pathways and other cellular processes as described in [1]. Many of the genes identified during the search for the molecular basis of PDB turned out, perhaps not unsurprisingly, to play important roles in key cellular pathways of osteoclasts. We will first focus on the early-onset

S.V. Reddy (Ed): Advances in Pathobiology and Management of Paget's Disease of Bone.
DOI: http://dx.doi.org/10.1016/B978-0-12-805083-5.00006-3

Paget diseases, describe the genes affected, their role, and discuss the pathways affected by mutations found in patients. We will then return to the more common classic PDB to see what lessons can be learned about pathogenetic mechanisms from these early-onset conditions.

EARLY-ONSET PAGETIC SYNDROMES

Familial expansile osteolysis (FEO; OMIM 174810), early onset Paget's disease (ePDB), and expansile skeletal hyperphosphatasia (ESH) present within the first 3 decades of life and are syndromes with skeletal features similar to classic PDB, but with subtle differences in their clinical phenotypes (reviewed and compared in [2]). As for classic PDB, bisphosphonate therapy forms the basis of therapeutic management for these syndromes [3], but skeletal deformities can be very severe and orthopedic intervention is often required. The diseases are inherited in an autosomal dominant manner and their molecular basis was identified as heterozygous tandem duplication insertion mutations within exon one of *TNFRSF11a*, encoding receptor activator of NFκB (RANK; as reviewed in [4]). The length of the duplication differs between the syndromes: 18 base pairs (6 amino acids) for FEO, 27 base pairs (9 amino acids) for ePDB, and 15 base pairs (5 amino acids) for ESH. All mutations occur within the signal peptide region of *TNFRSF11a*, and the specific base pair at which the duplication starts varies between syndromes but also within syndromes [5,6].

RANK

RANK is a type I transmembrane receptor and a member of the TNF receptor superfamily. The critical role for RANK in osteoclast formation, function, and survival is highlighted by the fact that:

- Patients with loss-of-function mutations in *TNFRSF11A* have osteopetrosis characterized by absence of osteoclasts ("osteoclast-poor" osteopetrosis; reviewed in [7]);
- Genetic deletion of RANK in mice leads to a severe osteopetrotic phenotype due to lack of osteoclast formation [8].
- Genetic deletion of RANK signaling pathway intermediates in mice leads to severe osteopetrotic phenotype due to lack of osteoclast formation (reviewed in [4]).

RANK signaling is activated by the interaction of RANK ligand (RANKL) with RANK and negatively regulated by osteoprotegerin

(OPG), a decoy receptor for RANKL, illustrated in Fig. 6.1 and described in more detail below. The binding of RANKL to RANK triggers a signaling cascade involving the recruitment of multiple factors and ultimately resulting in activation of NFκB. RANK itself does not have any kinase activity and so recruits TNF receptor associated factor 6 (TRAF6) to its C-terminal domain. TRAF6 is stabilized by p62, the gene product of SQSTM1 (discussed in detail in Chapter 5 Mutant SQSTM1/p62 Signaling in Paget's Disease of Bone) and activates downstream mediators NEMO and IKKα via K63-linked autoubiquitination. This results in the targeted phosphorylation, K48-linked ubiquitination, and subsequent degradation of IKBα which releases NFκB heterodimers for translocation to the nucleus and to regulate osteoclast-specific genes. This signaling cascade is illustrated in Chapter 5, Mutant SQSTM1/p62 Signaling in Paget's Disease of Bone.

In preclinical studies, the osteoclast phenotype associated with deletion of RANK is osteopetrosis, but the effect of increased RANK expression is less

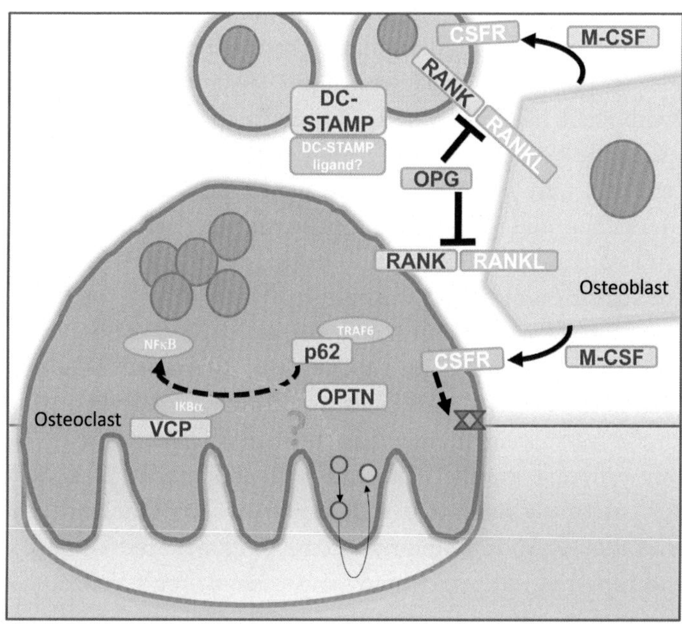

Figure 6.1 Schematic representation of the likely roles in osteoclasts for candidate genes implicated in classic Paget's disease of bone. Proteins identified in GWAS or through the study of monogenic syndromes with similar bone phenotypes are shown in red text. Interacting partners and/or key pathway intermediates are shown in white text.

clear. Mice overexpressing RANK in the monocyte lineage show increased numbers of osteoclasts in the jaw during tooth eruption and associated root canal remodeling [9]. The skeletal phenotype at other sites was not reported, but interestingly, monocytes from the transgenic animals did not yield larger numbers of osteoclasts in vitro, suggesting that the increase in osteoclasts in vivo may be through amplification of the premonocytic cells [9].

It was initially thought that hyperactivation of the RANK signaling pathway resulting in increased NFκB signaling, was the molecular mechanism causing early-onset Pagetic syndromes. However, a knockin mouse model of ePDB, the only animal model generated thus far for these conditions, showed characteristic osteolytic lesions only in heterozygous mice, while homozygous mice carrying the mutation died in utero as a result of severe osteopetrosis, caused by a complete absence of osteoclasts [10]. The reason for this unexpected finding became clear when the behavior of the mutant RANK proteins was analyzed in cell systems: all 3 insertion mutations resulted in a block in signal peptide cleavage, thereby preventing translocation of the translated RANK protein from the endoplasmic reticulum to the plasma membrane [11]. Instead of being expressed at the cell surface, the mutant proteins remained attached to the membrane of the endoplasmic reticulum where they were unable to interact with their ligand RANKL [11] and explaining the osteopetrotic phenotype in the homozygous ePDB mice. By contrast, when the mutant RANK proteins were coexpressed with wild-type RANK in cell systems, thereby modeling the genotype in patients who are all heterozygous, RANK was again detected at the plasma membrane and RANKL-dependent activation of NFκB was restored [12].

RANK proteins act as trimers and it is as yet unclear how mutant and wild-type proteins assemble in patient cells. In model cell systems, it appears that heterotrimeric molecules may form and that these are able to traffic to the plasma membrane. Such molecularly different receptors (containing different numbers of wild-type and mutant RANK monomers) may potentially interact in a different way to homotrimers consisting of wild-type RANK monomers only. Ongoing studies are trying to understand how the different homo- and heterotrimers that may exist in the heterozygous patient osteoclasts could prolong and/or increase RANK signaling resulting in the osteoclast pathology seen in vivo. Overall, it seems that the early-onset Pagetic syndromes caused by mutations in *TNFRSF11A* are part of a group of conditions in which defects in signal peptide cleavage disrupt normal protein function [13,14].

There remain many unanswered questions regarding these early-onset Pagetic syndromes and they are similar to those that remain open in classic PDB:

- Why are the conditions focal in nature?
- What are the environmental or genetic triggers for the development of specific lesions?
- What is the nature of the nuclear and cytoplasmic inclusions seen in osteoclasts in bone lesions?

Hormonal status and trauma have been suggested as possible triggers or facilitators of disease progression at a particular site [15], but so far there is no firm evidence for a causal effect.

Recently a new *TNFRSF11A* signal peptide mutation was reported in a patient with extreme panostotic high turnover bone disease, complicated by massive jaw tumors [16]. The molecular consequences of the mutation need further investigation. It is not clear at present whether this mutation is causal (and hence represents a new type of highly aggressive early onset PDB), or whether the tumors exacerbated the condition.

JUVENILE PAGET'S DISEASE

Juvenile Paget's disease (JPD; OMIM 239000) is a rare autosomal recessive condition featuring increased systemic bone remodeling resulting in weaker bones leading to fractures, presenting in young children and adolescents [17,18]. One recent case of JPD has been attributed to a heterozygous duplication mutation within the signal peptide region of *TNFRSF11A* [19], and polymorphisms within genes linked to late onset Paget's disease have been identified in a patient with mild JPD [20]. However, the condition is, on the whole, caused by deficiency of OPG through complete *TNFRSF11B* gene deletion or by loss-of-function mutations within *TNFRSF11B*.

Osteoprotegerin

OPG is secreted by osteoblasts as a decoy receptor for RANKL and hence controls RANKL-induced osteoclast activation by regulating the flux through the RANK signaling pathway. OPG acts as a dimer and seven different mutations have been described thus far, each directly responsible for the increased osteoclast activity seen in patients (Table 6.1). The mechanisms by which many of these mutations lead to OPG deficiency are reasonably well understood and summarized in [21] or as indicated.

Table 6.1 Summary of the genes and identified mutations or SNPs associated with early-onset Pagetic syndromes. Where the gene has also been associated with classic Paget's disease of bone this has been indicated. Please see chapter "Genetics of Paget's Disease of Bone" for a complete list of all genes associated with classic Paget's disease of bone

Gene (Protein)	Mutation/ SNP	Disease/syndrome
TNFRSF11A (RANK)	84dup18	Familial expansile osteolysis
	83dup18	
	75dup27	Early-onset Paget's disease
	78dup27	
	84dup15	Expansile skeletal hyperphosphatasia
	90dup12	Panostotic expansile osteolysis
	rs3018362	Classic Paget's disease of bone
TNFRSF11B (Osteoprotegerin)	Gene deletion	Juvenile Paget's disease
	686delG IVS3 + 19	
	T287C	
	G354A	
	638_640delGAC	
	T443C	
	965_967delTGA	
	969_970insTT130T > C	
	Deletion from intron 1226A > C	
	G1181C	Classic Paget's Disease
	C950T	
VCP (Valosin-containing-protein)	R155H (50% of patients)	Multisystem proteinopathy
	Twenty different missense mutations have been reported in total [29].	

- Gene deletion leads to complete OPG deficiency and a severe phenotype.
- A 20 base pair deletion leading to failure of splicing between exons 3 and 4 results in unstable mRNA and lack of OPG, also associated with a severe phenotype.

- A deletion of 3 base pairs in exon 3 is associated with relatively normal levels of circulating OPG. However, reduced affinity for RANKL results in reduced ability to inhibit osteoclast activity and an intermediate phenotype.
- A frameshift mutation within exon 5 leads to a truncated protein that cannot dimerize. Paradoxically, this mutation is associated with elevated levels of (dysfunctional) OPG and elevated levels of soluble RANKL, but with a mild phenotype.
- Missense mutations in exon 2 disrupt disulfide bonds and the tertiary structure of the ligand binding domain. These lead to severe phenotypes.
- Two substitution mutations: one replacing the initiation methionine [22] and one in the cysteine-rich domain responsible for OPG/RANKL interaction [23]. Both are associated with low circulating levels of OPG and a more severe phenotype.
- Deletion from intron 1 causing removal of exons 2–5 and loss of any ligand binding capacity resulting in a severe phenotype [24].
- Homozygous missense mutation in exon 2 likely to cause reduced affinity for RANKL and resulting in a mild to intermediate phenotype [24].

Clinical management of the skeletal pathology in JPD is by antiresorptive therapy. Calcitonin and bisphosphonates (Pamidronate, Ibandronate, and Zoledronate) have all been reported to improve clinical, biochemical, and radiographic parameters. OPG replacement therapy has been tried with some clinical success [25], but patients developed antibodies to synthetic OPG and this treatment is no longer available. Administration of anti-RANKL monoclonal antibody denosumab has also been reported in one patient [22]. In this patient, bone resorption and bone pain were more effectively controlled than with previous bisphosphonate treatment, but the patient suffered from severe hypocalcemia after the first administration of the drug, something also reported in a patient treated with Zoledronate [26]. Clearly, treatment regimens for these pediatric patients with excessive bone turnover need to be optimized and careful monitoring of serum calcium during treatment is required.

Multisystem Proteinopathy

Another syndromic form of Paget's disease is seen in the condition Inclusion Body Myopathy PDB and Frontotemporal Dementia [27], now referred to as multisystem proteinopathy (MSP) [28] since the ever-increasing range of patient phenotypes includes amyotrophic lateral sclerosis (ALS) and other motor neurone diseases. This rare autosomal dominant monogenic condition (OMIM 167320) affects three organ systems, although not every patient has symptoms in all three. Muscle weakness including ALS is most commonly seen (80% of patients), with PDB observed in about half and frontotemporal dementia in about a third of patients [29]. The onset of the muscle and bone disease is typically in the fourth to fifth decade with dementia from the sixth decade [29]. The disease is progressive and ultimately fatal. No disease-modifying treatments are available for the muscle disease, nor for the frontotemporal dementia. Patients with bone disease are treated using bisphosphonate therapy in the same way as patients with classic PDB [30].

Mutations in ubiquitously expressed gene for VCP located on chromosome 9p21.1–p12 are responsible for MSP [31]. Although the bone disease caused by mutations in *VCP* seems identical to that seen in classic PDB, it is only seen in the context of MSP; there is no genetic linkage to *VCP* in patients with sporadic or familial PDB [32]. To date more than 20 different *VCP* missense mutations have been identified in 37 affected families ([29], Table 6.1) with mutations located in multiple different domains of the protein.

Valosin-containing protein

VCP, also known as p97, or cdc48, is a highly expressed protein of 806 amino acids. VCP is a member of the type II AAA-ATPase gene superfamily which is highly conserved through evolution. It functions as a homohexamer. The protein interacts with more than 40 different cofactors, allowing it to take part in many and diverse cellular processes, for example in organelle formation, in cell cycle progression and in DNA repair. Important in the context of MSP is the role that VCP plays in protein degradation pathways (Fig. 6.2). Like p62, VCP has an ubiquitin binding domain and it assists in removing misfolded proteins from secretory pathways, including through facilitating retrograde transport out of the endoplasmic reticulum back to the cytoplasm and to the proteasome; a process called ERAD (endoplasmic reticulum-associated protein degradation). The precise ways in which the many different VCP mutations reported in MSP interfere with its function are not yet fully understood. Molecular modeling has shown that the mutations, although in different protein domains, affect a region at the interface between the N and D1

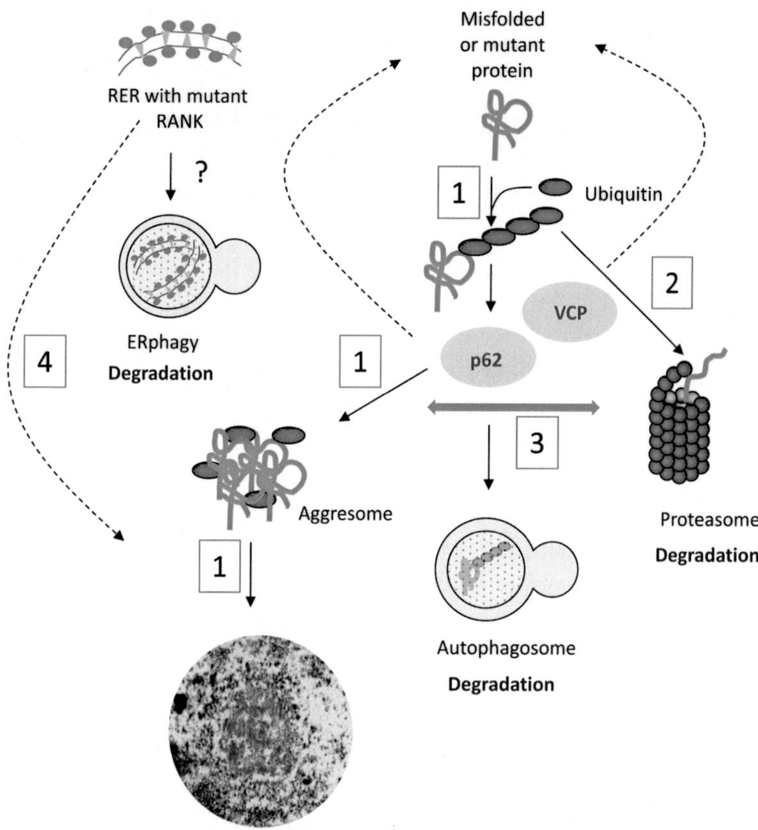

Figure 6.2 Schematic representation of the autophagy and proteasomal pathways illustrating how mutations seen in Pagetic diseases might cause protein accumulation and inclusion body formation (adapted from [60]). Please note that conclusive evidence for these pathways in patient osteoclasts is not yet available. (1) If p62 is mutated and hence inefficient in shuttling cargo to the autophagosomes, cytoplasmic aggregates may form. Since p62 is itself degraded by autophagy (see dotted lines), this degradation pathway is compromised even more and cytoplasmic aggregates may become aggresomes (visible structure) and inclusions. (2) Mutated VCP is less efficient in shuttling ubiquitinated substrates to the proteasome. (3) As the two pathways of protein degradation are linked, the presence of mutant VCP is likely to lead to inhibition of proteasomal degradation and a shift to autophagosomal degradation. This can again lead to stress on the autophagosomal system, formation of aggregates and ultimately inclusions. (4) We also hypothesize that RANK proteins with signal peptide mutations (FEO, ePDB and ESH), which render them unable to be released from the inner envelope of the ER, may lead to degradation of the dysfunctional ER by ER-phagy (discussed in [4]).

domains in the folded protein with conformational change leading to altered cofactor binding [33,34]. For some cofactors the change in conformation leads to reduced binding (eg, the most commonly seen mutation, R155H, reduces binding of the cofactor ubiquitin ligase E4B and CHMP5), however, for others it increases binding, while for yet another group there appears to be no change. The overall implications for VCP function therefore remain difficult to assess however some changes in cofactor binding have been associated with reduced VCP ATPase activity [35]. Interestingly, osteoclast-specific knockdown of CHMP5 results in a severe Pagetic phenotype (increased osteoclast and osteoblast activity) in mice, associated with reduced inhibition of NFκB activation [33]. This is possibly linked to the role of VCP in degrading specific substrates including IκB, a key component in the RANK signaling pathway ([36], Fig. 6.1).

The pathology of MSP has been most extensively studied in muscle and brain, with studies performed in patients, but also in transgenic or in knockin mouse models carrying the R155H or A232E mutations, and most recently in *Drosophila* models where the VCP homolog TER94 has been mutated [29]. In both animal models important features of the disease as seen in humans have been observed, such as muscle degeneration, neuronal and learning defects, and, in the mouse, bone disease [37]. These models thus offer in vivo systems for further exploration of the pathogenic mechanisms and for testing of new therapies such as recently reported for autophagy-modulating rapalogs [38].

Typical histological features of MSP are:

- Presence of rimmed vacuoles in muscle with inclusions containing ubiquitin and TAR-DNA binding protein-43 (TDP-43);
- Presence of ubiquitin- and TDP-43 containing inclusions in neurons.

There is no detailed information about the presence of inclusions in osteoclasts in bone, but given their presence in muscle in those patients with myopathy, it is expected that inclusions like those seen in classic PDB are present in those patients that have bone disease. The ultrastructural similarities of the inclusions in muscle in inclusion body myopathy with Paget's disease and frontotemporal dementia (IBMPFD) and those in osteoclasts in classic PDB have led to suggestions that both conditions may be part of the group of conformational disorders, a group that also contains several neuropathies and is associated with ER dysfunction through either ER stress or ER overload [39]. Similar to neurons, osteoclasts as postmitotic cells may be particularly sensitive to accumulation of misfolded proteins, which they cannot dilute through cell division.

MOLECULAR MECHANISMS LEADING TO EARLY-ONSET PAGETIC DISORDERS AND RELEVANCE FOR LATE-ONSET PDB

In Chapter 3 Genetics of Paget's Disease of Bone the genetic regions that have been associated with classic PDB (OMIM 602080; reviewed in [40]) were discussed. It has long been realized that the classic disease is genetically heterogeneous and through candidate gene, linkage, and latterly genome-wide association studies (GWAS) several candidate genes and genetic regions have been identified that may be causally associated with the disease [41–43]. Perhaps not surprisingly, these studies identified, amongst others, associations with *TNFRSF11A* and *TNFRSF11B*, two genes already known to be responsible for the early-onset Pagetic syndromes. A couple of other genes identified are similarly known as key players in regulation of osteoclast development, such as *CSF1* and *TM7S4*. Another gene, *OPTN*, is associated with many functions, including protein degradation, making tentative links to key roles of *SQSTM1* and *VCP*. So far, however, the only gene in which disease-causing mutations have been found in late onset disease is in *SQSTM1*, encoding the protein p62. We discuss briefly how molecular alterations in these genes, different from those changes already discussed in early-onset disease, might act and how the early-onset diseases may help identify key pathways that may be involved in late-onset disease.

CLASSIC PDB: ASSOCIATION WITH GENES INVOLVED IN RANK SIGNALING AND/OR OSTEOCLAST FORMATION

- *TNFRSF11A*

  The essential role of RANK for osteoclast development and function has been described above. The knowledge gained from FEO, ePDB, and ESH has illustrated that functional consequences of mutations in multimeric receptors in heterozygous patients may not be easily predictable. The genetic variants associated with classic PDB are downstream of *TNFRSF11A* and may not affect protein structure, but could positively affect levels of protein expression. Such overexpression may have an effect on early monocytic precursors as shown in studies in RANK transgenic mice [9], leading potentially to increases in osteoclast numbers upon stimulation of bone resorption. Such a mechanism may explain the increased sensitivity to pro-osteoclastogenic cytokines seen in patients.

- *TNFRSF11B*
  TNFRSF11B, encoding OPG, has also been described above. In mouse models, deletion of OPG results in severe osteoporosis [44] and patients with JPD have varying degrees of accelerated bone turnover, suggesting that aberrant expression or regulation of this protein would be associated with the increased osteoclast activation associated with classic PDB. Although *TNFRSF11B* was not identified in the GWAS for classic PDB, earlier studies in UK and Belgian population cohorts had identified risk haplotypes across *TNFRSF11B* only in women [45,46]. The molecular link between the associated SNPs and disease has not been studied in detail but the G1181C change results in a change from a positively charged lysine to an uncharged asparagine within the signal peptide of OPG and may therefore alter membrane insertion during posttranslational processing of the protein which could affect the release of OPG into the bone microenvironment [45].
- *CSF1*

CSF1 encodes macrophage colony stimulating factor (M-CSF), a cytokine critical for the differentiation of hematopoietic cells to the osteoclast lineage. M-CSF is produced by osteoblasts and stromal cells within the bone microenvironment and is essential, via binding to c-fms (encoded by *CSF1R*), to induce expression of RANK on osteoclast precursors. Other key functions for M-CSF in osteoclast development and activity include a permissive role in integrin signaling, increasing the affinity of β_3 integrin for ligand and stimulation of Rho family mediated cytoskeletal rearrangement (Fig. 6.1; reviewed in [47]). Differential splicing of exon 6 produces a membrane-bound or a secreted form of the glycoprotein [48]. M-CSF and RANKL then jointly drive differentiation of committed precursors toward terminally differentiated osteoclast precursors and induce expression of genes necessary for their fusion and the activity of mature osteoclasts (reviewed in [47]). *CSF1R*-knockout mouse models and naturally occurring mouse models with *CSF1* mutations have osteopetrosis, which can be rescued by administering recombinant M-CSF, or transgenic overexpression of the cytokine [48].

Surprisingly, to date there have been no reports of human bone disease associated with *CSFR1* or *CSF1* mutations, but three common genetic variants within the CSF1 gene have been associated with aggressive periodontitis, a condition that is characterized by early onset destruction of the alveolar bone [49]. Although there is, as yet, no clear association from population-based cohorts for a link between common variants within *CSF1* and development of late onset PDB, it is tempting to postulate that intronic SNPS may influence splicing and potentially alter the ratio of the membrane-bound versus the secreted form of the protein, the latter having been shown in mice to be specifically associated with pathological bone loss, such as after estrogen withdrawal in female mice [50]. Whether such mechanisms may be involved in the temporal nature (late onset) of the disease remains to be seen.

• *TM7S4*

TM7S4 encodes dendritic cell-specific transmembrane protein (DC-STAMP), a protein that regulates the fusion of osteoclast precursors to form multinucleated, resorbing cells [51]. This function was first demonstrated in knockout mouse models, and then by knockdown of DC-STAMP in human osteoclast cultures in vitro [52]. DC-STAMP expression is induced on osteoclast precursors by RANKL. To date, the DC-STAMP ligand has not been clearly identified, however it has been suggested that interaction of osteoclast precursors with the matricellular protein CCN2 via DC-STAMP upregulates osteoclast formation [53]. A role for DC-STAMP in PDB appears to make biological sense and the likely mechanism could be one of overexpression, or activation to lead to the increased size and multinuclearity of osteoclasts in patients.

CLASSIC PDB: GENES INVOLVED IN PROTEIN DEGRADATION PATHWAYS

• *OPTN*

OPTN encodes optineurin, first identified associated with glaucoma. Although the precise role for optineurin in osteoclasts has not been investigated, the functions of optineurin in other cell types (reviewed in [54]) suggest it could potentially regulate key processes in osteoclast formation, function, and survival, through negative regulation of NFκB activation; by preventing osteoclast apoptosis, or by regulating vesicular transport. Of particular interest in relation to protein degradation pathways is the role of OPTN in regulating the assembly of autophagosomes.

• *SQSTM1*

A multitude of mutations associated with SQSTM1/p62 ubiquitin associated (UBA) domain have been identified in patients with PDB. The functional role of mutant p62 and NFκβ activation is covered in detail in Chapter 5, Mutant SQSTM1/p62 Signaling in Paget's Disease of Bone.

PDB: A DISORDER OF PROTEIN CONFORMATION?

The remarkable similarities in inclusion bodies described in osteoclasts in late onset PDB, in FEO, in inclusion body myositis, and MSP has led to the hypothesis that PDB may be a disease of dysfunctional protein breakdown, leading to formation of protein aggregates and hence a conformational protein disease [55,56]. It remains difficult to understand how such a mechanism could lead to the upregulation of osteoclast activity, the hallmark of the Pagetic osteoclasts, as in general in conformational diseases cell death is the end result of prolonged protein aggregate accumulation. There is an alternative view suggesting that the inclusions represent viral nucleocapsid and evidence has been presented in cell and mouse models (discussed in Chapter 2: Viral Etiology of Paget's Disease of Bone) to show that paramyxoviral viral infection can induce an osteoclast phenotype with similarities to that seen in PDB. While it may be easier to understand how viral infection may upregulate osteoclast activity, the evidence from genetic, cell, animal, and human studies is pointing increasingly to a role for dysfunctional autophagy, possibly coupled with dysfunctional proteasomal degradation in PDB.

Key evidence for a causal role of autophagy/protein degradation in osteoclasts is:

- Presence of inclusion bodies in early-onset (FEO) and classic PDB;
- Presence of autophagy-related proteins as well as mutant proteins in these inclusions: p62 and ubiquitin in late-onset PDB; VCP, ubiquitin, and LC3 in muscle in MSP (reviewed in [56]).
- Inclusions are seen in cells that show no evidence of paramyxoviral presence [57].
- Studies in cell models expressing mutant forms of p62 and in absence of paramyxovirus show formation of inclusions identical in ultrastructural and immunohistochemical properties to those seen in patient osteoclasts [58].
- A mouse model with a knockin of the most common p62 mutation shows bone lesions with enlarged osteoclasts in the absence of viral infection and signs of deregulated autophagy in osteoclast precursors [59].

Fig. 6.2 shows the autophagy pathway and links with the proteasomal protein degradation pathway and indicates where p62 and VCP act. A putative role for optineurin is also shown. Inclusions in FEO and the other RANK-related early-onset diseases may find their origin in the need to recycle ER with uncleaved mutant RANK protein, a process that may involve ER-phagy (autophagic degradation of areas of ER) and could cause strain on overall protein degradation pathways. There is, however, as yet no direct evidence for this.

Acknowledgments

The authors wish to acknowledge grant support received from Arthritis Research UK (grants 13630; 19531; 20049), the Medical Research Council (G1000435), the Cunningham Trust and The Paget's Association.

REFERENCES

[1] Crockett JC, Rogers MJ, Coxon FP, Hocking LJ, Helfrich MH. Bone remodelling at a glance. J Cell Sci 2011;124(Pt 7):991–8.
[2] Takata S, Yasui N, Nakatsuka K, Ralston SH. Evolution of understanding of genetics of Paget's disease of bone and related diseases. J Bone Miner Metab 2004;22 (6):519–23.
[3] Riches PL, Imanishi Y, Nakatsuka K, Ralston SH. Clinical and biochemical response of TNFRSF11A-mediated early-onset familial Paget's disease to bisphosphonate therapy. Calcif Tissue Int 2008;83(4):272–5.
[4] Crockett JC, Mellis DJ, Scott DI, Helfrich MH. New knowledge on critical osteoclast formation and activation pathways from study of rare genetic diseases of osteoclasts: focus on the RANK/RANKL axis. Osteoporos Int 2011;22(1):1–20.
[5] Ke YH, Yue H, He JW, Liu YJ, Zhang ZL. Early onset Paget's disease of bone caused by a novel mutation (78dup27) of the TNFRSF11A gene in a Chinese family. Acta Pharmacol Sin 2009;30(8):1204–10.
[6] Johnson-Pais TL, Singer FR, Bone HG, McMurray CT, Hansen MF, Leach RJ. Identification of a novel tandem duplication in exon 1 of the TNFRSF11A gene in two unrelated patients with familial expansile osteolysis. J Bone Miner Res 2003;18 (2):376–80.
[7] Sobacchi C, Schulz A, Coxon FP, Villa A, Helfrich MH. Osteopetrosis: genetics, treatment and new insights into osteoclast function. Nat Rev Endocrinol 2013;9 (9):522–36.
[8] Dougall WC, Glaccum M, Charrier K, et al. RANK is essential for osteoclast and lymph node development. Genes Dev 1999;13(18):2412–24.
[9] Castaneda B, Simon Y, Jacques J, et al. Bone resorption control of tooth eruption and root morphogenesis: involvement of the receptor activator of NF-kappaB (RANK). J Cell Physiol 2011;226(1):74–85.
[10] Albagha OM, Rojas J, Van't Hof R, Dorin J, Ralston SH. Phenotypic characteristics of mice with an insertion mutation affecting the RANK signal peptide. Bone 2007;40:S148.
[11] Crockett JC, Mellis DJ, Shennan KI, et al. Signal peptide mutations in RANK prevent downstream activation of NF-kappaB. J Bone Miner Res 2011;26(8):1926–38.
[12] Mellis D, Duthie A, Clark S, Crockett JC. Investigating homozygous vs heterozygous expression of disease-associated receptor activator of NFkB mutations in vitro. Bone Abstracts 2013;1:PP233.
[13] Chan D, Ho MS, Cheah KS. Aberrant signal peptide cleavage of collagen X in Schmid metaphyseal chondrodysplasia. Implications for the molecular basis of the disease. J Biol Chem 2001;276(11):7992–7.
[14] Godi M, Mellone S, Petri A, et al. A recurrent signal peptide mutation in the growth hormone releasing hormone receptor with defective translocation to the cell

surface and isolated growth hormone deficiency. J Clin Endocrinol Metab 2009;94 (10):3939–47.
[15] Whyte MP, Reinus WR, Podgornik MN, Mills BG. Familial expansile osteolysis (excessive RANK effect) in a 5-generation American kindred. Medicine (Baltimore) 2002;81(2):101–21.
[16] Schafer AL, Mumm S, El-Sayed I, et al. Panostotic expansile bone disease with massive jaw tumor formation and a novel mutation in the signal peptide of RANK. J Bone Miner Res 2014;29(4):911–21.
[17] Whyte MP, Obrecht SE, Finnegan PM, Jones JL, Podgornik MN, McAlister WH, et al. Osteoprotegerin deficiency and juvenile Paget's disease. N Engl J Med 2002;347(3):175–84.
[18] Cundy T, Hegde M, Naot D, et al. A mutation in the gene TNFRSF11B encoding osteoprotegerin causes an idiopathic hyperphosphatasia phenotype. Hum Mol Genet 2002;11(18):2119–27.
[19] Whyte MP, Tau C, McAlister WH, et al. Juvenile Paget's disease with heterozygous duplication within TNFRSF11A encoding RANK. Bone 2014;68:153–61.
[20] Donath J, Speer G, Kosa JP, et al. Polymorphisms of CSF1 and TM7SF4 genes in a case of mild juvenile Paget's disease found using next-generation sequencing. Croat Med J 2015;56(2):145–51.
[21] Chong B, Hegde M, Fawkner M, et al. Idiopathic hyperphosphatasia and TNFRSF11B mutations: relationships between phenotype and genotype. J Bone Miner Res 2003;18(12):2095–104.
[22] Grasemann C, Schundeln MM, Hovel M, et al. Effects of RANK-ligand antibody (denosumab) treatment on bone turnover markers in a girl with Juvenile Paget's disease. J Clin Endocrinol Metab 2013;98(8):3121–6.
[23] Saki F, Karamizadeh Z, Nasirabadi S, Mumm S, McAlister WH, Whyte MP. Juvenile paget's disease in an Iranian kindred with vitamin D deficiency and novel homozygous TNFRSF11B mutation. J Bone Miner Res 2013;28(6):1501–8.
[24] Naot D, Choi A, Musson DS, et al. Novel homozygous mutations in the osteoprotegerin gene TNFRSF11B in two unrelated patients with juvenile Paget's disease. Bone 2014;68:6–10.
[25] Cundy T, Davidson J, Rutland MD, Stewart C, DePaoli AM. Recombinant osteoprotegerin for juvenile Paget's disease. N Engl J Med 2005;353(9):918–23.
[26] Polyzos SA, Anastasilakis AD, Litsas I, et al. Profound hypocalcemia following effective response to zoledronic acid treatment in a patient with juvenile Paget's disease. J Bone Miner Metab 2010;28(6):706–12.
[27] Kimonis VE, Kovach MJ, Waggoner B, et al. Clinical and molecular studies in a unique family with autosomal dominant limb-girdle muscular dystrophy and Paget disease of bone. Genet Med 2000;2(4):232–41.
[28] Benatar M, Wuu J, Fernandez C, et al. Motor neuron involvement in multisystem proteinopathy: implications for ALS. Neurology 2013;80(20):1874–80.
[29] Nalbandian A, Donkervoort S, Dec E, et al. The multiple faces of valosin-containing protein-associated diseases: inclusion body myopathy with Paget's disease of bone, frontotemporal dementia, and amyotrophic lateral sclerosis. J Mol Neurosci 2011;45(3):522–31.
[30] Kimonis V, Donkervoort S, Watts G. Inclusion body myopathy with Paget disease of bone and/or frontotemporal dementia. In: Pagon RA, Adam MP, Bird TD, Dolan CR, Fong CT, Stephens K, editors. GeneReviews. Seattle, WA: University of Washington; 2007.
[31] Watts GD, Wymer J, Kovach MJ, et al. Inclusion body myopathy associated with Paget disease of bone and frontotemporal dementia is caused by mutant valosin-containing protein. Nat Genet 2004;36(4):377–81.

[32] Lucas GJ, Mehta SG, Hocking LJ, et al. Evaluation of the role of Valosin-containing protein in the pathogenesis of familial and sporadic Paget's disease of bone. Bone 2006;38(2):280–5.
[33] Greenblatt MB, Park KH, Oh H, et al. CHMP5 controls bone turnover rates by dampening NF-kappaB activity in osteoclasts. J Exp Med 2015;212(8):1283–301.
[34] Ju JS, Weihl CC. Inclusion body myopathy, Paget's disease of the bone and fronto-temporal dementia: a disorder of autophagy. Hum Mol Genet 2010;19(R1):R38–45.
[35] Zhang X, Gui L, Zhang X, et al. Altered cofactor regulation with disease-associated p97/VCP mutations. Proc Natl Acad Sci U S A 2015;112(14):E1705–14.
[36] Dai RM, Chen E, Longo DL, Gorbea CM, Li CC. Involvement of valosin-containing protein, an ATPase Co-purified with IkappaBalpha and 26 S proteasome, in ubiquitin-proteasome-mediated degradation of IkappaBalpha. J Biol Chem 1998;273(6):3562–73.
[37] Badadani M, Nalbandian A, Watts GD, et al. VCP associated inclusion body myopathy and paget disease of bone knock-in mouse model exhibits tissue pathology typical of human disease. PLoS One 2010;5(10).
[38] Nalbandian A, Llewellyn KJ, Nguyen C, Yazdi PG, Kimonis VE. Rapamycin and chloroquine: the in vitro and in vivo effects of autophagy-modifying drugs show promising results in valosin containing protein multisystem proteinopathy. PLoS One 2015;10(4):e0122888.
[39] Roussel BD, Kruppa AJ, Miranda E, Crowther DC, Lomas DA, Marciniak SJ. Endoplasmic reticulum dysfunction in neurological disease. Lancet Neurol 2013;12(1):105–18.
[40] Ralston SH, Albagha OM. Genetic determinants of Paget's disease of bone. Ann N Y Acad Sci 2011;1240:53–60.
[41] Albagha OM, Visconti MR, Alonso N, et al. Genome-wide association study identifies variants at CSF1, OPTN and TNFRSF11A as genetic risk factors for Paget's disease of bone. Nat Genet 2010;42(6):520–4.
[42] Albagha OM, Wani SE, Visconti MR, et al. Genome-wide association identifies three new susceptibility loci for Paget's disease of bone. Nat Genet 2011;43(7):685–9.
[43] Chung PY, Van Hul W. Paget's disease of bone: evidence for complex pathogenetic interactions. Semin Arthritis Rheum 2012;41(5):619–41.
[44] Mizuno A, Amizuka N, Irie K, et al. Severe osteoporosis in mice lacking osteoclastogenesis inhibitory factor/osteoprotegerin. Biochem Biophys Res Commun 1998;247(3):610–15.
[45] Daroszewska A, Hocking LJ, McGuigan FE, et al. Susceptibility to Paget's disease of bone is influenced by a common polymorphic variant of osteoprotegerin. J Bone Miner Res 2004;19(9):1506–11.
[46] Beyens G, Daroszewska A, de Freitas F, et al. Identification of sex-specific associations between polymorphisms of the osteoprotegerin gene, TNFRSF11B, and Paget's disease of bone. J Bone Miner Res 2007;22(7):1062–71.
[47] Mellis DJ, Itzstein C, Helfrich MH, Crockett JC. The skeleton: a multi-functional complex organ: the role of key signalling pathways in osteoclast differentiation and in bone resorption. J Endocrinol 2011;211(2):131–43.
[48] Yao GQ, Wu JJ, Ovadia S, Troiano N, Sun BH, Insogna K. Targeted overexpression of the two colony-stimulating factor-1 isoforms in osteoblasts differentially affects bone loss in ovariectomized mice. Am J Physiol Endocrinol Metab 2009;296(4):E714–20.
[49] Rabello D, Soedarsono N, Kamei H, et al. CSF1 gene associated with aggressive periodontitis in the Japanese population. Biochem Biophys Res Commun 2006;347(3):791–6.

[50] Kimble RB, Srivastava S, Ross FP, Matayoshi A, Pacifici R. Estrogen deficiency increases the ability of stromal cells to support murine osteoclastogenesis via an interleukin-1and tumor necrosis factor-mediated stimulation of macrophage colony-stimulating factor production. J Biol Chem 1996;271(46):28890–7.
[51] Yagi M, Miyamoto T, Toyama Y, Suda T. Role of DC-STAMP in cellular fusion of osteoclasts and macrophage giant cells. J Bone Miner Metab 2006;24(5):355–8.
[52] Zeng Z, Zhang C, Chen J. Lentivirus-mediated RNA interference of DC-STAMP expression inhibits the fusion and resorptive activity of human osteoclasts. J Bone Miner Metab 2013;31(4):409–16.
[53] Nishida T, Emura K, Kubota S, Lyons KM, Takigawa M. CCN family 2/connective tissue growth factor (CCN2/CTGF) promotes osteoclastogenesis via induction of and interaction with dendritic cell-specific transmembrane protein (DC-STAMP). J Bone Miner Res 2011;26(2):351–63.
[54] Kachaner D, Genin P, Laplantine E, Weil R. Toward an integrative view of Optineurin functions. Cell Cycle 2012;11(15):2808–18.
[55] Agnati LF, Guidolin D, Woods AS, et al. A new interpretative paradigm for Conformational Protein Diseases. Curr Protein Pept Sci 2013;14(2):141–60.
[56] Hocking LJ, Whitehouse C, Helfrich MH. Autophagy: a new player in skeletal maintenance? J Bone Miner Res 2012;27(7):1439–47.
[57] Azzam E, Helfrich MH, Hocking L. Functional assessment of Paget's disease-causing mutations in sequestosome-1 (SQSTM1). Bone Abstracts 2013;1:493.
[58] Azzam E, Helfrich MH, Hocking L. Mutations in Sequestosome-1 result in inclusion body formation. Bone 2012;50:64.
[59] Daroszewska A, van't Hof RJ, Rojas JA, et al. A point mutation in the ubiquitin-associated domain of SQSTM1 is sufficient to cause a Paget's disease-like disorder in mice. Hum Mol Genet 2011;20(14):2734–44.
[60] Hocking LJ, Scott DI, Helfrich MH. Paget's disease of bone: a conformational disorder? Clin Laborat Internat 2008;3:7–9.

CHAPTER 7

Osteosarcoma in Paget's Disease of Bone

Margaret Seton[1] and Marc F. Hansen[2]
[1]Division of Rheumatology, Brigham & Women's Hospital, Boston, MA, United States
[2]Center for Molecular Medicine, University of Connecticut Health Center, Boston, MA, United States

INTRODUCTION

Pagetic osteosarcoma is a rare complication of Paget's disease of bone (PDB) [1].

- The association between Paget's disease and an increased risk of malignant transformation has been known since Sir James Paget first described the disease in 1876, in a paper entitled "On a Form of Chronic Inflammation of Bones (Osteitis Deformans)" [2]. In this paper, he wrote that "In 3 out of 5 well-marked cases that I have seen or read-of cancer appeared late in life; a remarkable proportion, possibly not more than might have occurred in accidental coincidences, yet suggesting careful inquiry." Later, he would capture more cancer deaths in the 23 patients he followed over the years, and bone and tumor registries would begin to publish pagetic osteosarcomas accounting for 5–30% of these late onset osteogenic bone cancers. These numbers vary depending on the volume of cases captured by the referral center reporting this rare cancer, and the ability to confirm the histology. What is consistent in the studies on pagetic osteosarcoma is as follows:
- White males are predominantly affected
- The peak age is the 7th–8th decades
- The incidence of malignant transformation is estimated to be 0.15–0.9% [3]
- The initial clinical presentation tends to be pain, swelling, and fracture
- The serum alkaline phosphatase is variably elevated
- Early radiographic findings often show an expanding lytic lesion in bone. Differentiation from PDB can be difficult in the absence of a soft tissue mass

S.V. Reddy (Ed): *Advances in Pathobiology and Management of Paget's Disease of Bone.*
DOI: http://dx.doi.org/10.1016/B978-0-12-805083-5.00007-5

- The histopathology in the majority of cases of osteosarcoma demonstrates stromal cell abnormalities, some degree of osteoid, and chaotic bone remodeling
- Outcomes for patients with pagetic osteosarcomas are poor, with 5-year survival rates of those in their 7th–8th decade reported as 12–17%. (http://seer.cancer.gov/statfacts/html/bones.html) [4,5]

EPIDEMIOLOGY

In 1957, Charles Porretta and colleagues at the Mayo Clinic reviewed the epidemiology of osteosarcoma in PDB in the English literature. Following Sir Paget's description of sarcoma arising in pagetic bone, Porretta described two other reports in 1878, and another case in 1894, which described the evolution of sarcoma in pagetic bone following fracture. This started a discussion of whether fracture through pathological bone might be permissive to the osteosarcoma. In fact trauma as causal to Paget's disease has been considered as an environmental determinant of disease, but its role in the expression of PDB or this rare complication of PDB remains hypothetical.

In Dr Porretta's paper, he identified 1753 patients with PDB in the medical records of the Mayo Clinic, of whom 16 were documented to have an osteosarcoma arising in pagetic bone. He calculated an incidence of 0.9%. In 1981, Wick and colleagues pooled these cases and extended the observation period from 1927 to 1977, identifying 3964 patients with PDB in records of the Mayo Clinic [6]. Of these, 38 were diagnosed with a pagetic osteosarcoma; they calculated a similar incidence rate. Analyzing the number of osteosarcomas seen during this time period, the authors found that pagetic osteosarcoma accounted for 3.1% of these, but >20% if one looked at cases in those >40 years of age.

Price in 1962 investigated the relationship between osteogenic sarcoma in the southwest of England and PDB. Drawing 87 cases from the Bristol Tumor Registry, he showed that 26 arose in association with PDB (30%). Further, he demonstrated that the elderly peak in osteosarcoma present in England was almost absent in Norway, a country in which PDB is rare [7]. This observation holds true for Asian nations, in which both PDB and elderly onset osteosarcoma are rare [8]. It is important to remember that estimates of the prevalence of osteosarcoma in the population of patients with PDB are skewed by the asymptomatic nature of this focal bone disease, and the size of a referral population on which conclusions are drawn.

Over the last 50 years or so, there is a sense that both the prevalence of PDB in a population and its severity have been declining in most nations studied; that the age of onset is later [9]; and that the proportion of PDB patients accounting for osteosarcomas in the elderly has diminished. This is supported by a study of osteosarcoma incidence and survival rates from 1973 to 2004 in the United States in which the incidence of osteosarcomas occurring >65 years was 4.2 per million ($n = 653$). Sixty-two cases of these cases in the elderly arose in pagetic bone (9.5%), occurring more often in men (1.58:1), with a peak age of 75 years. This cohort accounted for 19% of all osteosarcomas reported, with the decline in incidence over these years largely attributed to a decline in pagetic and secondary osteosarcomas [10]. This antedated the introduction of treatment for PDB in the form of bisphosphonates [11]. In fact many patients continue to present with pagetic osteosarcoma unaware of their underlying PDB.

The waning incidence of osteosarcomas arising in pagetic bone mirrors to some extent the decreasing prevalence of PDB in the population and the older age at presentation, but seems more pronounced [11]. Because osteosarcoma is so rare in the age-matched general population, this occurrence of pagetic osteosarcoma represents a several 1000-fold increase in risk over background [10–14]. There are isolated reports of familial clustering of osteosarcoma in Paget's disease; a linkage to a region of chromosome 18q in several families has been described [15–17].

CLINICAL PRESENTATION

Pagetic osteosarcomas tend to present with pain. Swelling around the bone and/or soft tissue mass are also common [14,18]. By radiographic imaging, the tumors frequently appear to be lytic lesions (Fig. 7.1). This lytic nature of Paget's disease explains the frequency of pathological fractures, which may mark the presentation of malignant transformation in bone. Elevated levels of alkaline phosphatase have been reported although the degree of elevation appears to be highly variable.

Initial reports suggested that pagetic osteosarcoma was more common in polyostotic Paget's disease [1,19], however, more recent reports suggests that there is no significant difference in incidence of pagetic osteosarcoma between the monostotic and polyostotic forms of Paget's disease [11,18,20]. Earlier studies had also proposed that malignant transformation

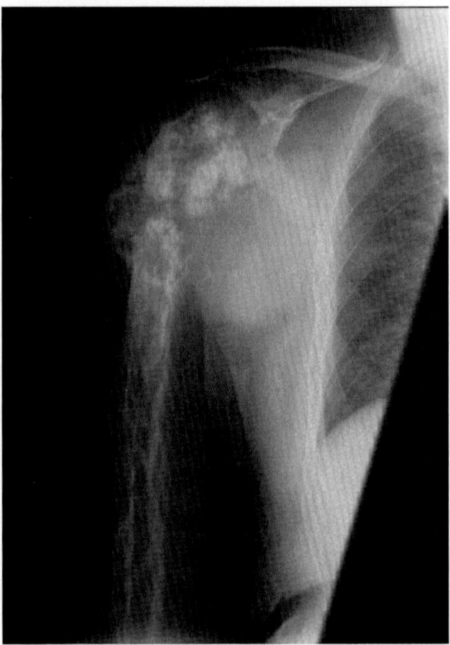

Figure 7.1 Radiogram of a pagetic osteosarcoma shows a destructive bone-forming lesion. Right shoulder of an elderly patient with an osteosarcoma arising in pagetic bone. Note the coarsened trabeculae, tunneled cortex, and remodeling of bone of the humerus that is classic of Paget's disease of bone. There is destruction of the proximal humerus by a soft tissue mass. *Radiograph courtesy of Dr Daniel I. Rosenthal, MD, Massachusetts General Hospital.*

resulted from a prolonged period of untreated Paget's disease. Several recent papers have questioned this assumption [18,20]. One study showed that 54% of patients developed osteosarcoma within 1 year of diagnosis while the remainder had a clinical history of Paget's disease that ranged from 16 months to 40 years with a mean of 15 years and a median of 10 [18] suggesting that the causes of tumorigenesis may not be simple.

The most common sites for pagetic osteosarcoma are the humerus, the pelvis, and femur [1,11,14,18,21]. For the most part, the anatomic distribution of pagetic osteosarcoma reflects that of the distribution of Paget's disease (Fig. 7.2), except that the spine is frequently affected by PDB but is a rare site for pagetic osteosarcoma [1,11,14,18,21]. Similarly, the humerus is less often affected in PDB but not an uncommon site for pagetic osteosarcoma [1,11,14,18,21]. Little is understood about the divergence of these patterns in two skeletal sites.

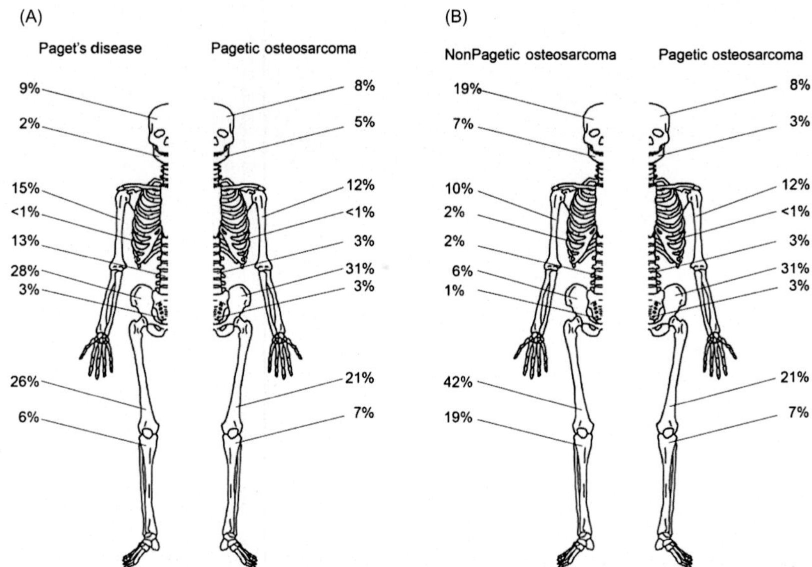

Figure 7.2 Skeletal Distribution of Pagetic osteosarcoma compared to (A) Paget's disease and (B) Nonpagetic osteosarcoma. Skeletal distributions of Paget's disease and pagetic osteosarcoma are based on an aggregation of samples reported in a number of published reports [1,11,14,18,21]. Skeletal distribution of nonpagetic osteosarcomas is based on [22]. Any differences in distribution frequencies between this figure and the published reports are the result of accumulation of fractional differences.

HISTOPATHOLOGY

Over 80% of the tumors associated with Paget's disease are osteosarcomas making it the most common malignancy associated with Paget's disease [14,18]. Other less common malignancies associated with Paget's disease include fibrosarcoma, malignant fibrous histiocytoma, chondrosarcoma, and giant cell tumor [18,23].

Most osteosarcomas that arise from Paget's disease are conventional, high-grade, intramedullary, lytic tumors with highly pleiomorphic cells [14,18]. The most common histological type was osteoblastic osteosarcoma followed by fibroblastic and chondroblastic [18]. The overall histological appearance of the tumors is consistent with an exaggerated form of the chaotic bone remodeling process found in Paget's disease (Fig. 7.3). The tumors are also characterized by the infiltration of osteoclast-like giant cells that are similar to those found in pagetic bone.

The tumors feature a high degree of cortical destruction and infiltration into the surrounding soft tissues [14,18]. Indeed, osteolysis is the

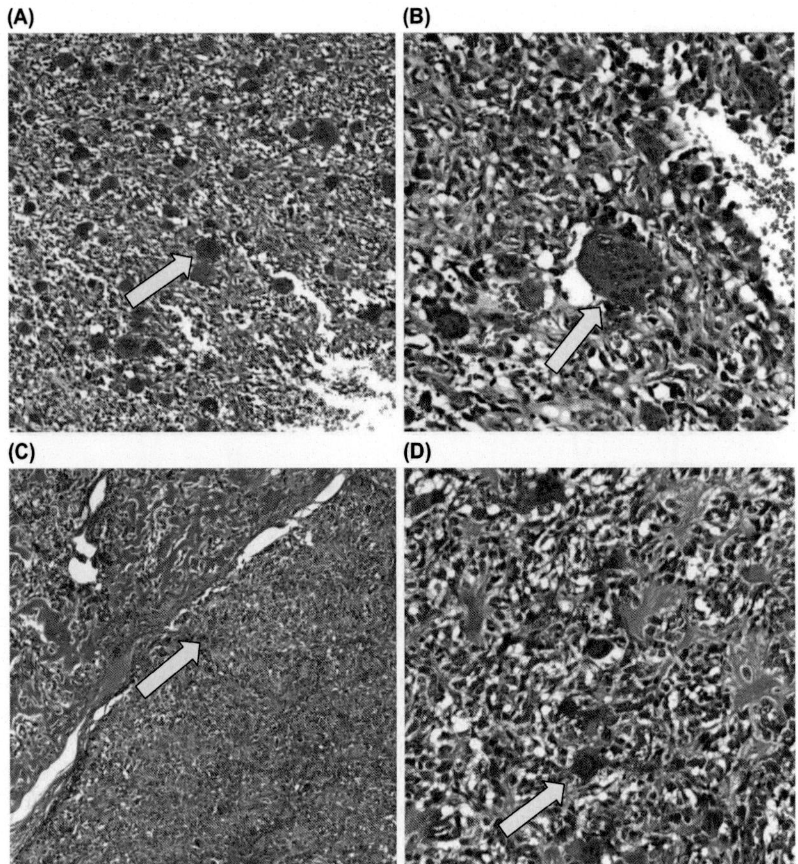

Figure 7.3 Histology of pagetic osteosarcoma showing infiltration of giant osteoclast-like cells. Arrows indicate examples of the giant osteoclast-like cells. A/C, Low magnification (40X nominal magnification); B/D, High magnification (100X nominal magnification).

major characteristic feature of pagetic osteosarcoma and only rarely do the tumors show intraosseus or extraosseus sclerosis [14,18]. Periosteal reaction, a characteristic feature of adolescent osteosarcoma is typically absent in the pagetic osteosarcoma.

TREATMENT AND PROGNOSIS

A multidisciplinary approach to treatment of adolescent osteosarcoma introduced in 1984 involving adjuvant chemotherapy and surgery has greatly improved the prognosis in adolescent osteosarcoma [24,25]. Unfortunately, this approach to treatment has not been as successful in pagetic osteosarcoma [1,10,18,26,27]. It has consistently been shown that pagetic osteosarcomas have a significantly worse prognosis than adolescent osteosarcoma [1,10,18,26,27]. Moreover, this prognosis has not changed despite the introduction of adjuvant chemotherapy for treatment [1,18]. In one study, the median survival for patients diagnosed before 1985 was 10 months while median survival for patients diagnosed after 1985 was 16 months [18]. In all reports, the 5-year survival for pagetic osteosarcoma has remained below 25% in contrast to the 5-year survival in adolescents, which has improved to over 70% [1,10,18,26,27].

There are several possible explanations for the observation that pagetic osteosarcoma has a significantly worse prognosis than adolescent osteosarcoma. One simple explanation is that the advanced age and generally poor health of Paget's disease patients could limit the aggressive use of chemotherapy [1,18,26–28]. Poor outcome is also compounded by the anatomic location of the pagetic tumors. A majority of pagetic osteosarcomas are located within the pelvis, proximal femur, and proximal humerus in contrast to adolescent osteosarcoma patients whose tumors occur more commonly in the distal femur and proximal tibia [18]. Another possibility is that the Paget's disease, with its attendant pain and bone malformation might mask early signs of malignant transformation [30]. It is also possible that this delay in diagnosis might result in larger and more advanced tumors upon final detection. This is partly supported by the report that the percentage of pagetic osteosarcoma patients with initial Stage III presentation (27%) exceeds that of adolescent patients (13%) [18]. Another possibility is that the frequent presence of giant osteoclast-like cells within the tumor [18] may also play a role in the poorer prognosis, allowing the tumors to make a more rapid transition to a metastatic phenotype [31,32]. Finally, pagetic osteosarcoma tumors typically have a very high degree of vascularity [18], which would also permit a more rapid onset of metastasis.

Taken together, these confounding factors would all have a worsening effect on the outcome of pagetic osteosarcoma when compared to the relative success of treatment of adolescent osteosarcoma. The need for improved treatment of pagetic osteosarcoma will require a better understanding of the critical events that control the process of malignant transformation in the pagetic lesion. By understanding the details of deregulated signaling pathways, we may gain new targets for therapeutic intervention in this rare but deadly complication of Paget's disease.

THE PROGRESSION FROM NORMAL BONE TO PAGET'S DISEASE TO PAGETIC OSTEOSARCOMA

Our understanding of the genetic etiology of Paget's disease is currently evolving [33–35]. It was initially thought that mutations and environmental signals in the osteoclast and circulating precursors created a permissive environment for upregulation of remodeling that led to the development of Paget's disease [14,36]. However, there is evidence that the osteoblastic and stromal cells within the microenvironment of the evolving Paget's disease may also play a significant role in the etiology of Paget's disease [14,37–39]. Our understanding of the etiology of pagetic osteosarcoma supports this notion of a role for the osteoblastic lineage cells within the developing lesion.

There are three general phases in the progression of Paget's disease [36]: the initial or osteolytic phase in which enhanced osteoclastic activity is observed. It is during this phase that the characteristic pagetic osteoclasts, with their dramatically increased size and numbers of nuclei appear. This is followed by a mixed lytic/sclerotic phase in which rapid remodeling of the bone takes place with increases of both osteoblastic and osteoclastic activity. During this period, the initial bone resorption is gradually taken over by bone formation and overgrowth. The erratic remodeling process results in irregular cortical bone formation, marked by tunneling osteoclasts and deformation of bone that are visible on plain films. The histopathology demonstrates a mosaic pattern of cement lines, as the lamellar bone becomes disorganized by the deposition of woven bone. Bone trabeculae thicken, but the architecture of bone remains abnormal. Over time, this accelerated bone remodeling can give way to more dense, biochemically quiet bone that remains structurally unsound.

Pagetic osteosarcomas appear to arise in metabolically active bone in both monostotic and polyostotic Paget's disease, predominantly during the mixed lytic/sclerotic phase of Paget's disease [14]. One possible explanation for this timing is that this period is marked by rapid cell division in the pagetic osteoblasts. This rapid cell division could result in an increased frequency of somatic mutations and give rise to changes that would lead to malignant transformation. That somatic mutations in genes such as *SQSTM1* can occur within the tissues of the pagetic lesions has been shown [40], but what the exact nature of the genetic alterations needed to complete the malignant transformation are remains to be defined. A recent report suggests treatment with bisphosphonates may affect malignant transformation of pagetic bone [20], but this is a small observational study so the published results generate a hypothesis that needs to be corroborated.

Therefore, pagetic osteosarcomas would appear to represent a diversion in the normal progression of PDB [14]. This diversion would likely represent an accumulation of somatic mutations that would be distinct from those involved in the progression of the disease that would give rise to the biochemically quiet bone typical of late-stage PDB. Comparative analysis of the osteoblasts from different stages of PDB with the tumor cells of the pagetic osteosarcoma would be informative in understanding the process of malignant transformation.

GENES DIFFERENTIALLY EXPRESSED IN PAGET'S DISEASE AND PAGETIC OSTEOSARCOMA

In the progression from normal bone to Paget's disease to pagetic osteosarcoma there are generally six possible patterns of differentially expressed gene. These are shown in Fig. 7.4. In classes I and II, the genes are similarly expressed in both Paget's disease and pagetic osteosarcoma and would likely represent changes that occurred during the initial PDB disease process. In classes III and IV, there are differential changes in expression only in the pagetic osteosarcoma and it is likely that these would represent genes that are important in the malignant transformation. Finally, in classes V and VI, there are genes whose expression shows progressive changes from normal to Paget's disease to pagetic osteosarcoma. These would represent genes that may be important in the progression of the disease.

Several studies have compared gene expression between osteoblasts from pagetic osteoblasts and normal osteoblasts [39,41–43] as well as compared normal osteoclasts to pagetic osteoclasts [44]. This has yielded a set of genes that appear to be important in a number of cell function and signaling pathways. Curiously, these genes appeared to be from a number of distinct but interrelated signaling pathways (Fig. 7.5).

Use of the DAVID Functional Annotation Bioinformatics database (david.abcc.ncifcrf.gov/) [49,50] identified a number of KEGG signaling pathways [51] known to be associated with these genes, including the

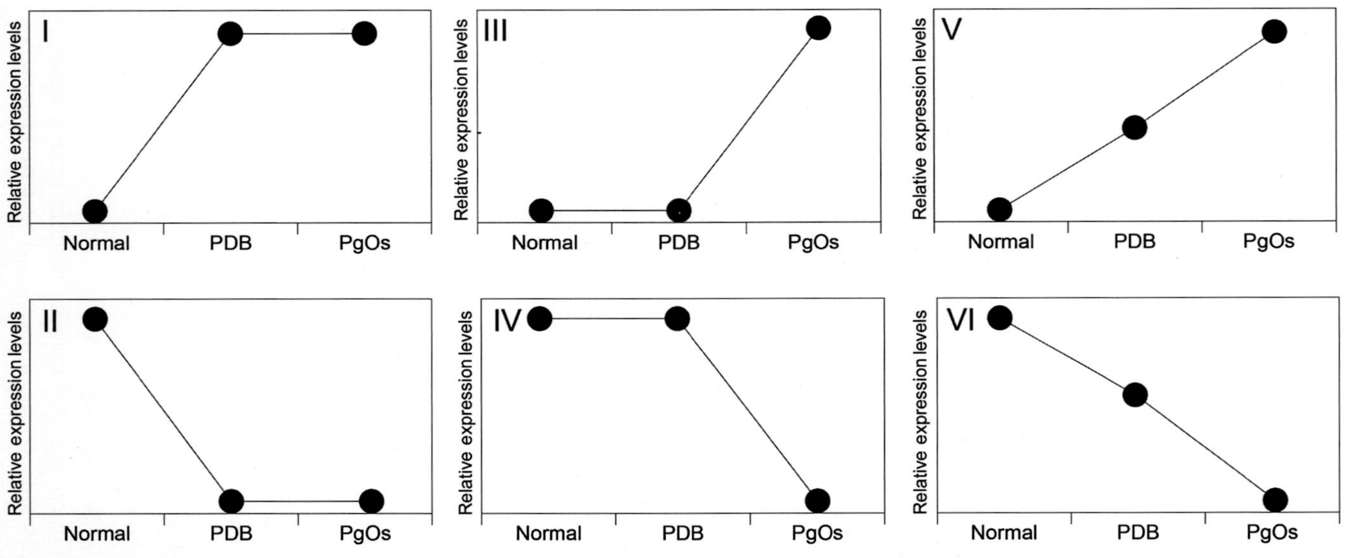

Figure 7.4 Potential classes of gene expression patterns in progression from normal osteoblast to Paget's disease osteoblast to pagetic osteosarcoma. Classes are based on changes in relative expression levels between normal osteoblasts (Normal), osteoblasts from pagetic lesions (PDB), and tumor cells from pagetic osteosarcomas (PgOs).

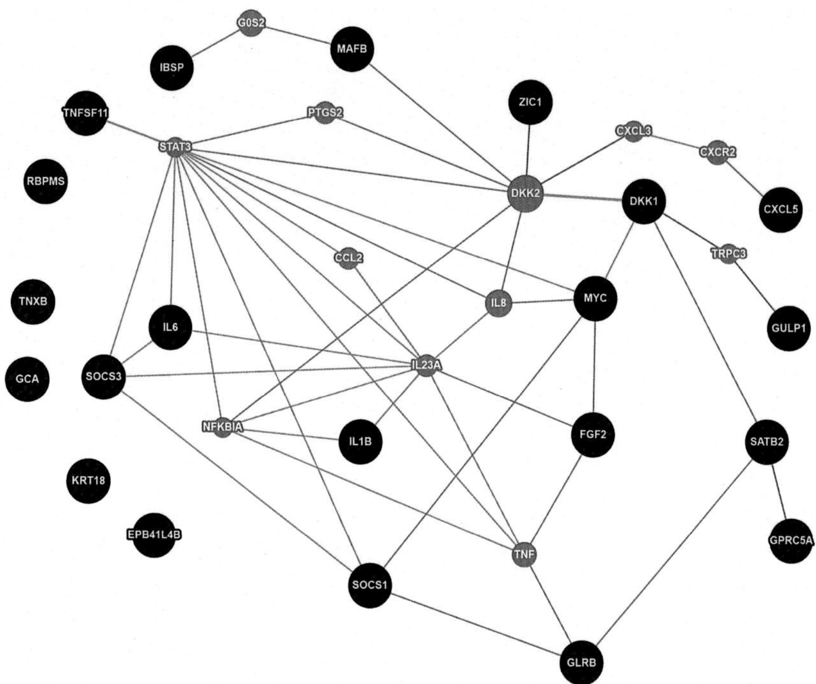

Figure 7.5 Gene interactions between the genes identified as differentially expressed between normal osteoblasts and pagetic osteoblasts and pagetic osteosarcoma tumor cells. Gene association patterns were drawn using GeneMania [45]. Large dark circles represent differentially expressed genes identified in previous studies [39,41–43,46] while small gray circles represent linker genes between the differentially expressed genes. Red lines indicate known signaling pathway interactions [47]. Purple lines indicate known genetic interactions [48]. Genes with no lines were not found to have known interactions with the other genes in the set.

NF-kB, Jak-STAT, Wnt, and MAPK signaling pathways, as well as the ECM-receptor interaction pathway, suggesting that multiple pathways have to be altered to give rise to Paget's disease. While receptor activator of NFκB (RANK)-RANK ligand (RANKL) signaling is clearly implicated in malignancy and cancer metastasis in breast and prostate cancer [52], there appeared to be a divergence as to whether RANKL expression was increased or decreased in the pagetic osteoblasts [39,41–43], suggesting that RANK signaling may be only one of several alternative sets of pathways involved in PDB and ultimately pagetic osteosarcoma.

Differential gene expression in pagetic osteosarcoma consistent with the Class III or IV pattern of expression has been reported in only one study that showed upregulation of the *MYC* gene in pagetic osteosarcoma relative to pagetic and normal osteoblasts [46].

A small sample set comparing differential gene expression analysis between normal, Paget's disease osteoblasts and pagetic osteosarcoma cells showed no difference in levels of expression between the pagetic osteoblasts and pagetic osteosarcoma tumor cells for some of the genes from the published studies [39,41–43] suggesting that these genes found in these previous reports were of the Class I and II patterns of gene expression and reflect the PDB disease process initiation rather than the tumorigenic transformation (unpublished data). MYC was found to be upregulated and analysis suggested that the majority of differentially expressed genes in the pagetic osteosarcomas came from the KEGG Pathways in the Cancer signaling pathway [51] (unpublished results).

Unsurprisingly, genes shown to be differentially expressed in pagetic osteoclasts relative to normal osteoclasts [44] showed no correlation of expression with the differentially expressed genes in the normal and pagetic osteoblasts [39,41–43] or the tumor cells from the pagetic osteosarcomas (unpublished data), consistent with the hypothesis that the pagetic osteosarcomas did not arise from these hematopoietic origin cells. Gene expression in the giant osteoclast-like cells that infiltrate the pagetic osteosarcomas have not as yet been examined although this would be an interesting comparison with the giant osteoclast-like cells that infiltrate the pagetic bone to see if there are tumor-specific changes in these infiltrating cells.

A number of studies have examined differential gene expression in adolescent osteosarcoma and several gene signatures have been correlated with adolescent osteosarcoma tumor progression and chemotherapy resistance [32,53–57]. Curiously, there also appears to be little concordance between the genetic signatures in these studies [32,53–57] suggesting that these tumors may also be very complicated in their etiology. However, a few similarities have been found between PDB and adolescent and pagetic osteosarcomas. Both PDB and adolescent osteosarcomas upregulate DKK1 expression [39,58,59] while MYC is upregulated in both adolescent and pagetic osteosarcoma [46,60,61]. Further analysis will be required to determine whether there are fundamental differences between adolescent and pagetic osteosarcoma, which reflect the differences in response to chemotherapy treatment that are observed between the two types of osteosarcoma.

Acknowledgments

The authors would like to thank Dr Daniel I. Rosenthal for providing the radiograph in Fig. 7.1 and Tracy Root and Christa Veno for administrative support. This work was supported in part by a grant (PR100793) from the Department of Defense Congressionally Directed Medical Research Program Peer Reviewed Medical Research Program.

REFERENCES

[1] Paget S. On a form of chronic inflammation of bones (osteitis deformans). Medical Chir Trans 1876;LX:1.
[2] Mankin HJ, Hornicek FJ. Paget's sarcoma: a historical and outcome review. Clin Orthop Relat Res 2005;438:97–102.
[3] Schajowicz F, Santini Araujo E, Berenstein M. Sarcoma complicating Paget's disease of bone. A clinicopathological study of 62 cases. J Bone Joint Surg Br 1983;65 (3):299–307.
[4] Porretta CA, Dahlin DC, Janes JM. Sarcoma in Paget's Disease of bone. J Bone Joint Surg 1957;13–14.
[5] Howlader N, Noone A, Krapcho M, et al. <http://seer.cancer.gov/csr/1975_2010/> SEER cancer statistics review, 1975–2010. Bethesda, MD: National Cancer Institute; 2013.
[6] Wick MR, Siegal GP, Unni KK, McLeod RA, Greditzer III HG. Sarcomas of bone complicating osteitis deformans (Paget's disease): fifty years' experience. Am J Surg Pathol 1981;5(1):47–59.
[7] Price CH. Osteogenic sarcoma; an analysis of the age and sex incidence. Br J Cancer 1955;9(4):558–74.
[8] Nishida Y, Isu K, Ueda T, et al. Osteosarcoma in the elderly over 60 years: a multicenter study by the Japanese Musculoskeletal Oncology Group. J Surg Oncol 2009;100(1):48–54.
[9] Corral-Gudino L, Borao-Cengotita-Bengoa M, Del Pino-Montes J, Ralston S. Epidemiology of Paget's disease of bone: a systematic review and meta-analysis of secular changes. Bone 2013;55(2):347–52.
[10] Mirabello L, Troisi RJ, Savage SA. Osteosarcoma incidence and survival rates from 1973 to 2004: data from the Surveillance, Epidemiology, and End Results Program. Cancer 2009;115(7):1531–43.
[11] Mangham DC, Davie MW, Grimer RJ. Sarcoma arising in Paget's disease of bone: declining incidence and increasing age at presentation. Bone 2009;44 (3):431–6.
[12] Mirabello L, Troisi RJ, Savage SA. International osteosarcoma incidence patterns in children and adolescents, middle ages and elderly persons. Int J Cancer 2009;125 (1):229–34.
[13] Grimer RJ, Cannon SR, Taminiau AM, et al. Osteosarcoma over the age of forty. Eur J Cancer 2003;39(2):157–63.
[14] Hansen MF, Seton M, Merchant A. Osteosarcoma in Paget's disease of bone. J Bone Miner Res 2006;21(Suppl. 2):P58–63.
[15] Nassar VH, Gravanis MB. Familial osteogenic sarcoma occurring in pagetoid bone. Am J Clin Pathol 1981;76(2):235–9.
[16] Wu RK, Trumble TE, Ruwe PA. Familial incidence of Paget's disease and secondary osteogenic sarcoma. A report of three cases from a single family. Clin Orthop Relat Res 1991;265:306–9.

[17] Mcnairn JD, Damron TA, Landas SK, Ambrose JL, Shrimpton AE. Inheritance of osteosarcoma and Paget's disease of bone: a familial loss of heterozygosity study. J Mol Diagn 2001;3(4):171–7.

[18] Deyrup AT, Montag AG, Inwards CY, Xu Z, Swee RG, Krishnan Unni K. Sarcomas arising in Paget disease of bone: a clinicopathologic analysis of 70 cases. Arch Pathol Lab Med 2007;131(6):942–6.

[19] Hansen MF, Nellissery MJ, Bhatia P. Common mechanisms of osteosarcoma and Paget's disease. J Bone Miner Res 1999;14(Suppl. 2):39–44.

[20] Zati A, Bilotta TW. Degeneration of Paget's disease into sarcoma: clinical and therapeutic influencing factors. Chir Organi Mov 2008;92(1):33–7.

[21] Seitz S, Priemel M, Zustin J, et al. Paget's disease of bone: histologic analysis of 754 patients. J Bone Miner Res 2009;24(1):62–9.

[22] Unni KK. Dahlin's bone tumors: general aspects and data on 11,087 cases. Philadelphia, PA: Lippincott-Raven; 1996.

[23] Horvai A, Unni KK. Premalignant conditions of bone. J Orthop Sci 2006;11 (4):412–23.

[24] Gill J, Ahluwalia MK, Geller D, Gorlick R. New targets and approaches in osteosarcoma. Pharmacol Ther 2013;137(1):89–99.

[25] Anninga JK, Gelderblom H, Fiocco M, et al. Chemotherapeutic adjuvant treatment for osteosarcoma: where do we stand? Eur J Cancer 2011;47(16):2431–45.

[26] Longhi A, Errani C, Gonzales-Arabio D, Ferrari C, Mercuri M. Osteosarcoma in patients older than 65 years. J Clin Oncol 2008;26(33):5368–73.

[27] Ruggieri P, Calabro T, Montalti M, Mercuri M. The role of surgery and adjuvants to survival in Pagetic osteosarcoma. Clin Orthop Relat Res 2010;468(11):2962–8.

[28] Seton M, Moses AM, Bode RK, Schwartz C. Paget's disease of bone: the skeletal distribution, complications and quality of life as perceived by patients. Bone 2011;48 (2):281–5.

[29] Bone HG. Nonmalignant complications of Paget's disease. J Bone Miner Res 2006;21(Suppl. 2):P64–8.

[30] Carter CJ, Ward WG. Osteosarcoma diagnostic delay associated with alendronate-induced pain relief. J Surg Orthop Adv 2012;21(3):165–9.

[31] Endo-Munoz L, Evdokiou A, Saunders NA. The role of osteoclasts and tumour-associated macrophages in osteosarcoma metastasis. Biochim Biophys Acta 2012;1826(2):434–42.

[32] Mintz MB, Sowers R, Brown KM, et al. An expression signature classifies chemotherapy-resistant pediatric osteosarcoma. Cancer Res 2005;65(5):1748–54.

[33] Roodman GD. Insights into the pathogenesis of Paget's disease. Ann N Y Acad Sci 2010;1192:176–80.

[34] Ralston SH, Layfield R. Pathogenesis of Paget disease of bone. Calcif Tissue Int 2012;91(2):97–113.

[35] Chung PY, Van Hul W. Paget's disease of bone: evidence for complex pathogenetic interactions. Semin Arthritis Rheum 2012;41(5):619–41.

[36] Siris ES, Roodman GD. Paget's disease of bone. In: Rosen CJ, editor. Primer on the metabolic bone diseases and disorders of mineral metabolism. *8th ed.* Ames, IA: John Wiley & Sons, Inc; 2013. p. 659–68.

[37] Singer FR, Leach RJ. Bone: do all Paget disease risk genes incriminate the osteoclast? Nat Rev Rheumatol 2010;6(9):502–3.

[38] Menaa C, Reddy SV, Kurihara N, et al. Enhanced RANK ligand expression and responsivity of bone marrow cells in Paget's disease of bone. J Clin Invest 2000;105 (12):1833–8.

[39] Naot D, Bava U, Matthews B, et al. Differential gene expression in cultured osteoblasts and bone marrow stromal cells from patients with Paget's disease of bone. J Bone Miner Res 2007;22(2):298–309.

[40] Merchant A, Smielewska M, Patel N, et al. Somatic mutations in SQSTM1 detected in affected tissues from patients with sporadic Paget's disease of bone. J Bone Miner Res 2009;24(3):484–94.

[41] Sundaram K, Rao DS, Ries WL, Reddy SV. CXCL5 stimulation of RANK ligand expression in Paget's disease of bone. Lab Invest 2013;93(4):472–9.

[42] Sundaram K, Senn J, Reddy SV. SOCS-1/3 participation in FGF-2 signaling to modulate RANK ligand expression in paget's disease of bone. J Cell Biochem 2013;114(9):2032–8.

[43] Sundaram K, Senn J, Yuvaraj S, Rao DS, Reddy SV. FGF-2 stimulation of RANK ligand expression in Paget's disease of bone. Mol Endocrinol 2009;23(9):1445–54.

[44] Michou L, Chamoux E, Couture J, Morissette J, Brown JP, Roux S. Gene expression profile in osteoclasts from patients with Paget's disease of bone. Bone 2010;46 (3):598–603.

[45] Warde-Farley D, Donaldson SL, Comes O, et al. The GeneMANIA prediction server: biological network integration for gene prioritization and predicting gene function. Nucl Acids Res 2010;38(Web Server issue):W214–20.

[46] Ueda T, Healey JH, Huvos AG, Ladanyi M. Amplification of the MYC gene in osteosarcoma secondary to Paget's disease of bone. Sarcoma 1997;1(3–4):131–4.

[47] Wu G, Feng X, Stein L. A human functional protein interaction network and its application to cancer data analysis. Genome Biol 2010;11(5):R53.

[48] Lin A, Wang RT, Ahn S, Park CC, Smith DJ. A genome-wide map of human genetic interactions inferred from radiation hybrid genotypes. Genome Res 2010;20 (8):1122–32.

[49] Huang Da W, Sherman BT, Lempicki RA. Systematic and integrative analysis of large gene lists using DAVID bioinformatics resources. Nat Protoc 2009;4(1):44–57.

[50] Huang Da W, Sherman BT, Lempicki RA. Bioinformatics enrichment tools: paths toward the comprehensive functional analysis of large gene lists. Nucl Acids Res 2009;37(1):1–13.

[51] Kanehisa M, Goto S. KEGG: kyoto encyclopedia of genes and genomes. Nucl Acids Res 2000;28(1):27–30.

[52] Dougall WC, Chaisson M. The RANK/RANKL/OPG triad in cancer-induced bone diseases. Cancer Metastasis Rev 2006;25(4):541–9.

[53] Borys D, Canter RJ, Hoch B, et al. P16 expression predicts necrotic response among patients with osteosarcoma receiving neoadjuvant chemotherapy. Hum Pathol 2012;43(11):1948–54.

[54] Horvai AE, Roy R, Borys D, O'donnell RJ. Regulators of skeletal development: a cluster analysis of 206 bone tumors reveals diagnostically useful markers. Mod Pathol 2012;25(11):1452–61.

[55] Man TK, Chintagumpala M, Visvanathan J, et al. Expression profiles of osteosarcoma that can predict response to chemotherapy. Cancer Res 2005;65(18):8142–50.

[56] Suehara Y, Kubota D, Kikuta K, Kaneko K, Kawai A, Kondo T. Discovery of biomarkers for osteosarcoma by proteomics approaches. Sarcoma 2012;2012:425636.

[57] Flores RJ, Li Y, Yu A, et al. A systems biology approach reveals common metastatic pathways in osteosarcoma. BMC Syst Biol 2012;6:50.

[58] Lee N, Smolarz AJ, Olson S, et al. A potential role for Dkk-1 in the pathogenesis of osteosarcoma predicts novel diagnostic and treatment strategies. Br J Cancer 2007;97 (11):1552–9.

[59] Marshall MJ, Evans SF, Sharp CA, Powell DE, Mccarthy HS, Davie MW. Increased circulating Dickkopf-1 in Paget's disease of bone. Clin Biochem 2009;42 (10–11):965–9.
[60] Shimizu T, Ishikawa T, Sugihara E, et al. c-MYC overexpression with loss of Ink4a/Arf transforms bone marrow stromal cells into osteosarcoma accompanied by loss of adipogenesis. Oncogene 2010;29(42):5687–99.
[61] Han G, Wang Y, Bi W. C-Myc overexpression promotes osteosarcoma cell invasion via activation of MEK-ERK pathway. Oncol Res 2012;20(4):149–56.

CHAPTER 8

Paget's Disease of Bone: Prognosis and Complications

Laëtitia Michou and Jacques P. Brown
Division of Rheumatology, Department of Medicine, CHU de Québec-Université Laval, Quebec City, QC, Canada

INTRODUCTION

Paget's disease of bone (PDB) is the second most frequent metabolic bone disorder after osteoporosis. The prevalence of PDB increases with age, affecting up to 3% of adults over 55 years of age. The high prevalence of PDB, previously reported in Lancashire (England) and in New Zealand, may be related to environmental and genetic factors, since both factors have been implicated in the pathogenesis of PDB. The secular declining prevalence and severity of PDB observed in the British population suggests that PDB is at least somewhat regulated by environmental factors. In support of a rural link to PDB, the region of Campania (Italy) was recently reported as a high prevalence area with increased severity and neoplastic degeneration of pagetic bones. Although frequently asymptomatic, about 30% of patients with PDB continue to experience disabilities due to bone pain, osteoarthritis secondary to bone deformities adjacent to weight-bearing joints, fractures, or nerve root compression. Sarcoma arising in PDB has tended to be less frequent in recent years, but the most severe complication of PDB can still be a presenting feature of this disease.

PROGNOSIS OF PAGET'S DISEASE OF BONE

Morbidity and Quality of Life

Morbidity in patients with PDB is mostly related to skeletal and nonskeletal complications attributable to PDB. The focal increases in bone turnover which characterizes PDB, resulting in abnormal bone architecture, weakened bone strength, and increased bone vasculature, largely explain the pathogenesis of mechanical, vascular, and metabolic complications.

S.V. Reddy (Ed): Advances in Pathobiology and Management of Paget's Disease of Bone.
DOI: http://dx.doi.org/10.1016/B978-0-12-805083-5.00008-7

Table 8.1 Frequencies of the most common complications of Paget's disease of bone in different countries

Country	USA	USA	UK	UK	France	Italy
References	[2]	[8]	[7]	[17]	[4]	[38]
Number of patients, *n*	202	236	2465	1324	446	147
Bone pain, %	47.5	41.9	66.7	46.7	99.7	NA
Bone deformity, %	36	7.6	9.2	35.9	27.2	NA
Fracture, %	14	9.7	7.9	39.1	10.8	13.6
Neurological complication, %	29	9.3	NA	NA	16.3	NA
Headache, %	10	NA	NA	NA	62.7	10.2
Hearing loss, %	20	61.4	6.9	22.3	52.6	13.6
Osteoarthritis, %	39	72.6	14.3	NA	97.8	45.6
Cardiovascular complication, %	NA	NA	NA	NA	10	21.8
Osteosarcoma, %	NA	0.4	0.3	NA	0.2	0

NA, not available.

These complications are reviewed in detail below, and the most common complications of the disease, in different countries with high prevalence of PDB, are presented in Table 8.1.

In a survey sent to 2000 people randomly selected from the Paget's Foundation mailing list, 47% of participants ($n = 958$) have reported feelings of depression, 42% said that their health was fair or poor, and only 21% reported very good or excellent quality of life [1]. The most frequent physical complications, as reported by participants who were long-time sufferers of PDB, were hearing loss (37%), bowed limbs (31%), leg length discrepancies (25%), fractures (19%), and enlarged head (17%). In the New England registry for PDB, the quality of life assessment allowed the authors to show that 44% of the 202 participating patients reported reduced physical activity, 32% needed to use chronic pain medications, and 25% needed to use a cane or walker [2]. Reduced self-care or depression was infrequently reported in this cohort (7% or below). Recently, a survey, performed in 285 participants of the New England registry for PDB, showed that compared to the general population, participants had lower levels of physical health, as determined by the 12-item Short-Form self-questionnaire (SF-12), and a slightly better mental component score [3]. Eighty-nine percent of participants reported complications of PDB, such as arthritis (48%), deformity (36%), nerve injury or chronic back pain (28%), hearing loss (22%), fractures (17%), problems with vision (14%), headache (13%), and joint replacement

(10%). Radiographic investigations confirmed that patients were aware of the presence of a disease complication, in particular bone deformity, fracture, and joint replacement, but were less correlative when headache or hearing loss was reported. In the ESOPE study (Epidemiology and Socioeconomics of PDB—a study among rheumatologists in France), the quality of life, evaluated in 387 patients with PDB by the use of the SF-36, was found to be significantly decreased in comparison to the general population in France aged 65–74 years and older than 74 years [4]. The authors reported that all eight SF-36 subscores were significantly worse in men than in women with PDB, in particular the mental health, the physical functioning, the vitality, the general health perceptions, and the social functioning. The quality of life and its clinical determinants were also studied in the 1324 patients with PDB who participated to the PRISM study, a randomized comparative trial of intensive versus symptomatic treatment for PDB [5]. The physical component summary score was significantly reduced in PDB patients versus an expected score from a normal population, and the mental component summary score was also significantly decreased but to a lesser degree. The greatest reduction in the SF-36 components was for the physical functioning, the bodily pain, the role physical, the role emotional, the social functioning, and the general health. For the bone pain due to PDB, previous bisphosphonate therapy and increasing age were found to be negative predictors of the SF-36 physical summary score in PDB. More recently, the analysis of the subgroup of 737 participants from the PRISM trial and for whom the *Sequestosome1 (SQSTM1)* mutation status was known, reported a significantly reduced SF-36 physical summary score in carriers of a *SQSTM1* mutation, which represents 10% of this cohort [6]. The authors concluded there is an increased disease severity in *SQSTM1* mutation carriers, based on a higher frequency of orthopedic surgery in patients who were carriers of a mutation (26.2% in carriers vs 16.1% in noncarriers, $p = 0.02$), a more common use of bisphosphonate therapy (86.3% vs 75.2%, $p < 0.01$), and a higher frequency of fractures (12.5% vs 5.3%, $p = 0.01$), although most of these fractures occurred in nonpagetic bones.

Mortality

The mortality of patients with PDB reported in the General Practice Research Database (GPRD) in England and Wales, after 5 years of follow up, was 32.7% in the patient group ($n = 2465$) and 28.0% in the control group ($n = 7395$), which represents a relative risk of 1.4 (1.1–1.4) [7].

The three most frequent causes of death were diseases of the circulatory system (37.9%), cancers (21.8%), and diseases of the respiratory system (20.9%). The relative risk of these three causes of death was significantly higher in the group with PDB than in the control group, relative risk of 1.5 (1.3–1.7), 1.8 (1.5–2.2), and 1.3 (1.1–1.6), respectively. In the population-based inception cohort of Olmsted County (Minnesota), patients with PDB were followed for 3408 person-years with a median of 13.4 years [8]. In comparison to residents of this county with the same age and sex distribution, the standardized mortality ratios (SMRs), in residents with PDB first diagnosed in 1950–1994, were not significantly increased for all causes of death (SMR = 0.97 (0.84–1.11)). The survival was better than expected since 10 years after the diagnosis of PDB, 62% of patients were still alive versus 57% expected. The men had significantly better survival (59% alive vs 52% expected) and the women had a trend toward better survival (66% alive vs 63% expected). The most frequent causes of death were diseases of the circulatory system (45%), cancers (19%), and diseases of the respiratory system (12%), but the SMR for these causes of death were not significantly increased. The authors found several clinical features of PDB that were significantly associated with an increased risk of death using an univariate model, but after adjusting for the population survival differences, no clinical risk factors remained associated with an increased risk of death in patients with PDB.

Impact of Pharmacological Treatment of PDB on the Prognosis

The pharmacological treatment of PDB, mainly represented by bisphosphonates, is classically indicated to prevent future complications in pagetic bones. Although the impact of bisphosphonates was demonstrated to be very effective to treat pagetic bone pain [8], their role in the prevention of complications, such as osteoarthritis, fracture, hearing loss, or other neurological complications, is less convincing in the literature [9]. In a long-term study, secondary osteoarthritis was more frequently reported in pagetic patients (62%) who had only a decrease in serum total alkaline phosphatase (sTALP) than those (33%) who had normal sTALP following bisphosphonate therapy [10]. Since it is always very difficult for clinicians to assess the respective role of pagetic bone pain and pain due to secondary osteoarthritis, the use of bisphosphonates in every case of pain arising close to a pagetic site can be considered as a reasonable strategy [11]. Bisphosphonates are indicated for all patients with active PDB, even if they are asymptomatic. These treatments are also indicated in the prevention of future complications, in particular for patients who have an involvement of long bones to decrease bowing deformities, an extensive skull involvement to prevent hearing loss, a vertebral pagetic involvement due to the risk of neurological complications, and in case of pagetic bones adjacent to weight-bearing joints to decrease the risk of secondary osteoarthritis [12,13]. Since current therapies improve radiographic osteolytic lesions [14] and allow normal lamellar bone deposition [15], it is likely that associated complications could be prevented if treatment is administered at an early stage [9,10,16]. In the PRISM study [17], intensive bisphosphonate therapy was not found to be effective on quality of life, bone pain, or clinical complications, such as fracture and osteoarthritis, in comparison to symptomatic treatment. These results may be explained by limitations in the design of this study [16,18], such as a treatment given late in the disease process, a possible inadequate primary endpoint (clinical fracture at any site instead of pain, or fracture in pagetic bone), a too small sample size and a too short observational period. Then the initiation of bisphosphonate therapy at an early stage of PDB should be more important to prevent future complications than the potency of the drug itself.

BONE COMPLICATIONS

Two-thirds of patients with PDB report pain, which is a very common clinical symptom of PDB. In up to a third of symptomatic patients, the pain can be attributed to degenerative joint disease [19], which often represents a complication of the disease. Patients with lower segment PDB such as affecting the lumbar spine, pelvis, or lower limbs had difficulty in determining the source of their pain between bone pain and joint pain. Pain associated with PDB tended to be less severe in patients with coexistent osteoarthritis or pagetic arthropathy, and less responsive to bisphosphonate therapy. The relationship of joint pain to joint movement or weight-bearing might be helpful to exclude the bone origin of the pain, as bone pain is expected to be mild to moderate in severity and also to be present at rest [13]. Bone pain attributed to PDB may be due to occurrence of stress fractures, to increased vascularity of bone, or may originate from the periosteum which may be stretched in weight-bearing of long bones. Normalization of blood flow in the affected bone with bisphosphonate therapy may influence pain relief [20]. In a recently published systematic review, bone pain was reported to occur in 52.2% of patients and was the most common presenting feature [21]. Bone deformity is also a classical complication of PDB, reported in an average of 30% of patients in different cohorts (Table 8.1) and in 21.5% of patients in a systematic review [21]. Anterior or lateral bowing of tibias or femurs is typical. In the spine, bowing may lead to a kyphosis and in the hip, protusio acetabuli may occur. Severe bone deformity may lead to intractable pain, limitation of motion and function, dysmorphic appearance, and the mechanical overload of the neighboring joints contribute to the development of severe degenerative joint disease [22]. Corrective osteotomy may be indicated to treat symptomatic patients with disabling deformity without degenerative joint disease. In candidates for arthroplasty with high degree of complexity of the bone deformity, corrective osteotomy at the time of arthroplasty and prior to joint replacement may be necessary. Corrective osteotomy was reported to be effective at providing pain relief, improvement of function, and satisfaction with cosmetic appearance of the limb. In a small case series of corrective osteotomies in patients with PDB, a higher prevalence of complications was observed following intramedullary nailing and external fixation [22] and the time to union of diaphyseal osteotomies was longer than in metaphyseal osteotomies. Pathological fractures or fractures of pagetic bone, which may be the first symptom of the disease, has been reported in 10–30% of patients [20]. Fractures of the long bones are more frequent at the mixed and osteoblastic stages of the disease. Union tends to be delayed in the osteoblastic and sclerotic phases, and nonunions in diseased bone are frequent. Partial or incomplete stress fractures, which are predisposing factors to complete fractures, are mostly observed on the tension side of long bones, such as in the subtrochanteric region. These insufficiency fractures appear as linear cortical radiolucent areas on the convex surface of long bones, and are also called "banana fractures" [23]. At the osteoblastic or sclerotic stages, in particular in the case of bone deformity, a prophylactic osteotomy and intramedullary stabilization is recommended. The overall fracture risk among patients with PDB, excluding fractures through pagetic bone, was not significantly increased in the population-based cohort of Olmsted County (standardized incidence ratio of 1.2 (0.9–1.4)) [24]. However, the authors reported a significant increase in risk of subsequent vertebral and rib fractures, but not for proximal femur or distal forearm. Forestier's disease or diffuse idiopathic skeletal hyperostosis (DISH) has been reported in 14–30% of patients with PDB [20]. DISH should not be confused with focal Pagetic bone formation or ankylosing spondylitis, which may coexist with PDB. Pagetic tissue may invade the hyperostotic lesions of DISH and transform them into pagetic exostoses, which further progresses into vertebral ankylosis. Periodontal complications due to PDB affecting the mandible or maxilla represent another bone complication of the disease, which accounts for 15% of cases [25]. Common dental complications are malocclusion, teeth mobility or loosening, root resorption, hypercementosis, excessive bleeding on extraction, osteomyelitis, infected gums, and poorly fitting dentures. Due to poor bone quality associated with pagetic bone, this disease, when affecting the jaws, is considered as a relative contraindication to dental implants.

SECONDARY OSTEOARTHRITIS

Osteoarthritis secondary to deformities adjacent to weight-bearing joints is a common complication of PDB, resulting from altered biomechanics across abnormal bones and joints leading to cartilaginous and osseous degeneration [23]. Erosion of the subchondral bone may lead to collapse of the articular cartilage. Bone expansion and bone deformity may also contribute to secondary osteoarthritis by incongruity of the articular cartilage [20]. The hip and the knee are the more frequently affected sites. Deformities such as coxa vara, femoral bowing, acetabular protusio, and bone enlargement may contribute to pagetic arthropathy at the hip [26] (Fig. 8.1). Pagetic arthropathy may require bisphosphonate treatment to control the disease activity, and medical treatment of osteoarthritis which relies mainly on antalgic or anti-inflammatory drugs, joint infiltrations, and physical activity. In the most severe cases, total hip arthroplasty may be helpful for pain relief, but the potential risk of loss of implant in the long term has been raised [26]. Adequate control of PDB by the use of bisphosphonate has been shown to decrease the risk of implant loosening, and this treatment also contributes to the decrease of intraoperative blood loss. The spine is the second most commonly affected site of PDB, which leads to low back pain and spinal stenosis. Back pain in PDB has been frequently attributed to coexisting osteoarthritis. Indeed, pagetic facet arthropathy highly contributes to back pain as well as spinal stenosis [20].

NEOPLASTIC DEGENERATION

The most severe but rare complication of PDB, malignant transformation to pagetic sarcoma, occurs in about 0.3% of patients. Sarcoma arising in

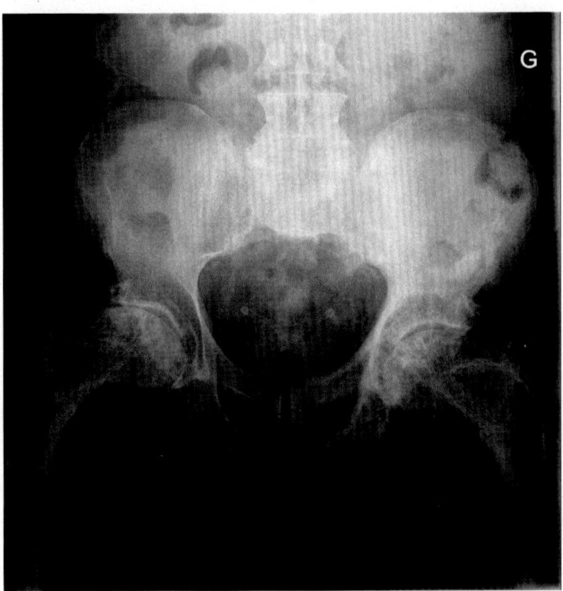

Figure 8.1 Pagetic arthropathy at both hips with typical deformities of both femoral necks leading to coxa vara and femoral bowing.

PDB tends to be less frequent in recent years, but can still be a presenting feature of the disease [27]. This malignant transformation may occur even if the disease is not so active. In addition, a higher number of affected bones is not a predictor of sarcoma occurrence. In a clinicopathologic analysis of 70 cases, pagetic sarcoma tended to occur in older men (mean age 66 years), predominating in the axial skeleton in particular in the pelvis, within patients with an average duration of the disease of 15 years [28]. Eighty-eight percent of these neoplasms were osteosarcomas, ie, with at least focal osteoid production (61% osteoblastic, 31% fibroblastic, and 8% chondroblastic), five cases were malignant fibrous histiocytomas and three cases were fibrosarcomas, all tumors being of high grade. The prognosis remains poor in presence of a pagetic sarcoma with a 5-year survival rate of 10%, the survival ranging from 1 month to 20 years. Teriparatide should not be prescribed for patients at increased baseline risk of osteosarcoma such as PDB. This complication is reviewed in detail in Chapter 7, "Osteosarcoma in Paget's Disease of Bone".

One must also keep in mind that elderly patients with preexisting PDB may frequently develop nonsarcomatous malignancies, such as metastatic carcinoma, which are more likely to occur due to the hypervascularity of the pagetic bone, as well as myeloma or lymphoma [29]. Benign tumors such as giant cell tumor may occur, although rarely reported in association with PDB. Giant cell tumors are then more frequent in patients with a polyostotic involvement, and occur in an older age group and are more common in the skull and facial bones. Finally, other diagnoses should be considered in the differential diagnosis of a tumor-like lesion in a patient with PDB, in particular active PDB and occult fractures, pseudosarcoma, postimmobilization lysis, and drug-induced osteomalacia [29].

NEUROLOGICAL COMPLICATIONS

The overgrowth or fractures of pagetic bone in the case of involvement of the skull and of one or more vertebrae may lead to central and peripheral nervous system complications, by direct compression of neural tissues or due to ischemia in relation with a vascular steal phenomenon [30]. All neurological structures, brain, spinal cord, and peripheral nerves, including cranial nerves, may be affected due to their close anatomical proximity to bone. Various neurological symptoms have been reported in patients with PDB, such as headache, dementia, brain stem, cerebellar dysfunction, cranial neuropathies, myelopathy, cauda equina syndrome, and radiculopathies [30]. Headache is frequently reported in patients with PDB (Table 8.1). The pagetic involvement of the skull may lead to severe headache, frequently in the occipital region, and is classically aggravated by coughing, sneezing, or straining. Pagetic osteosarcoma of the skull has been reported in the literature. This complication should be suspected in the presence of a partially fluctuant and locally painful skull mass associated with a rapid neurological deterioration. The softening of the skull base may lead to basilar invagination and further obstruction of the cerebrospinal fluid through basilar cisterns. The ventricular enlargement is associated with gait difficulties, incontinence, and dementia, which is the classical triad of normal pressure hydrocephalus. Dementia in PDB may also be caused by direct compression of the cerebral hemispheres. Therapeutic options are represented by surgical decompression, ventriculo-peritoneal shunt insertion, and medical treatment (mainly bisphosphonates). Other encephalic complications of PDB have been reported, such as compressive lesions due to ossification of extradural structures, hydrocephalic parkinsonism, epilepsy, and amyotrophic lateral sclerosis-like syndrome [30].

Cranial nerves compression, in particular of the olfactory and auditory nerves, are frequent in PDB. The optic nerve may also be affected, leading to diminished vision or blindness, retinal hemorrhage, choroiditis, optic atrophy, and papilloedema [30]. The intrinsic complications reported in PDB are corneal opacities, cataract, angioid streaks, and disciform macular degeneration [31]. Angioid streaks, which are observed in up to 15% of patients, should be recognized since they produce sight-threatening subretinal neovascular membranes, the latter being treatable. Other ocular complications are due to compression: papilloedema, optic atrophy, extraocular muscle palsies, exophthalmia, and nasolacrimal duct obstruction [31]. Facial nerve compression and trigeminal neuralgia have also been reported, leading to hemifacial spasm or facial paresis [30]. Hearing loss is a very common complication of PDB when the skull is involved (Table 8.1) and deafness was present in 8.9% of patients in a recent meta-analysis [21]. The mechanism of the sensorineural hearing loss in PDB is complex and may include compression of auditory nerve, vascular shunt, air-bone gap caused by stiffness in soft tissue elements of the middle ear, epitympanic spurs, or proliferation of fibrous tissue adjacent to ossicles [32]. The strong correlation between the bone mineral density of the cochlear capsule and air-bone gap now supports a possible alteration of the acoustical mechanisms of the ear more than a pathology of the ossicular chain [32]. Finally, the lower cranial nerves may be involved in the case of basilar invagination, leading to clinical symptoms, such as dysarthria, hoarseness, muscle atrophy (sternocleidomastoid, trapezius or tongue), fasciculation, and weakness [30].

The spine is affected in about half of patients with PDB, leading frequently to neurological deficits, including affection of the spinal cord, cauda equina, or nerve roots [33]. One-third of patients with PDB have clinical symptoms of spinal stenosis [20]. Compression fracture of the pagetic vertebral body may be associated with retropulsion of bone into the spinal canal, possibly leading to spinal stenosis in particular in the lumbar region. Spinal stenosis may also result from compressive myelopathy by bone overgrowth, ossification of epidural fat, or pagetic facet arthropathy [33]. In addition, noncompressive myelopathy may occur due to a vascular steal phenomenon. Spinal cord compression has been reported at the foramen magnum due to basilar invagination as a cause of quadriplegia, which can lead to formation of syringomyelia [20]. Cord or cauda equina compression may occur secondary to pagetic ossification of the extradural fat and ligamentum flavum adjacent to vertebrae affected by PDB [33]. Entrapment of the sciatic nerve may occur between an enlarged ischium and the lesser trochanter or between the abnormal ilium and piriformis muscle [23]. The treatment of spinal complications of PDB is difficult due to the involvement at multiple levels and the hypervascularity of bone with risk of bleeding [30]. This treatment relies mostly on medical treatment with bisphosphonate followed rarely by decompressive surgery.

CARDIOVASCULAR COMPLICATIONS

PDB involves the cardiovascular system by an increased incidence of calcific valvular disease and other endocardial calcifications, and a propensity for generalized atherosclerosis. In an autopsy series, aortic stenosis was found in 24% of the 27 patients with severe PDB versus 3.5% of the 201 controls ($p < 0.01$), whereas the prevalence of aortic stenosis in cases with PDB was similar to controls [34]. In a radiographic study of 42 patients with PDB and 36 controls, 52.4% of patients had arteriosclerotic calcification versus 30.6% of controls [35]. The patients with PDB also had more medial arterial calcification than controls and these calcifications were longer and thicker. In this study, patients with PDB were not reported to have more vascular complications, such as cerebrovascular accidents, coronary insufficiency, or distal arteritis, than controls. Since cardiac output increases with increasing extent of PDB, high-output heart failure is a theoretical complication of PDB, although very uncommon [13].

OTHER COMPLICATIONS

Several metabolic complications of PDB are well-known, such as an overproduction of parathyroid hormone (PTH) which is reported in 12–18% of patients with PDB [36]. A PDB-associated secondary hyperparathyroidism is more frequently observed than the true association between PDB and a primary hyperparathyroidism. High levels of PTH may drive responsive pagetic osteoclasts to levels of bone-resorbing activity that can exceed their intrinsic augmented states, leading to a pagetic hyperparathyroid syndrome [36]. This syndrome may be a consequence of increased calcium demands during periods of active new bone formation. Hypercalcemia is an unusual complication, classically occurring after immobilization [13]. Hypercalciuria and renal stones formation have also been uncommonly reported. Finally, PDB has been reported to be associated with hyperuricemia [13], with an increased incidence of gout and pseudogout [20], as well as with Peyronie's disease [37], the latter being more likely to be a disease association than a complication of PDB.

Disclosures

L. Michou is Scientific advisor for Merck, BMS, and Eli Lilly; on Speakers bureau: Actavis, Amgen, Eli Lilly, Novartis, Abbvie, and BMS; and has received Congress invitations by Amgen and Eli Lilly; and has received in kind kits for bone remodeling markers measurement from Roche Diagnostics Canada.

J.P. Brown is Scientific advisor for Amgen, Eli Lilly, and Merck; on Speakers bureau for Amgen, Eli Lilly; has received Congress invitations by Amgen and Eli Lilly; and has received Research grants from Amgen, Actavis, Eli Lilly, Merck, Novartis, and Takeda.

REFERENCES

[1] Gold DT, Boisture J, Shipp KM, Pieper CF, Lyles KW. Paget's disease of bone and quality of life. J Bone Miner Res 1996;11(12):1897–904.
[2] Seton M, Choi HK, Hansen MF, Sebaldt RJ, Cooper C. Analysis of environmental factors in familial versus sporadic Paget's disease of bone—the New England Registry for Paget's Disease of Bone. J Bone Miner Res 2003;18(8):1519–24.
[3] Seton M, Moses AM, Bode RK, Schwartz C. Paget's disease of bone: the skeletal distribution, complications and quality of life as perceived by patients. Bone 2011;48(2):281–5.
[4] Saraux A, Brun-Strang C, Mimaud V, Vigneron AM, Lafuma A. Epidemiology, impact, management, and cost of Paget's disease of bone in France. Joint Bone Spine 2007;74(1):90–5.
[5] Langston AL, Campbell MK, Fraser WD, Maclennan G, Selby P, Ralston SH. Clinical determinants of quality of life in Paget's disease of bone. Calcif Tissue Int 2007;80(1):1–9.
[6] Visconti MR, Langston AL, Alonso N, et al. Mutations of SQSTM1 are associated with severity and clinical outcome in paget disease of bone. J Bone Miner Res 2010;25(11):2368–73.
[7] van Staa TP, Selby P, Leufkens HG, Lyles K, Sprafka JM, Cooper C. Incidence and natural history of Paget's disease of bone in England and Wales. J Bone Miner Res 2002;17(3):465–71.
[8] Wermers RA, Tiegs RD, Atkinson EJ, Achenbach SJ, Melton 3rd LJ. Morbidity and mortality associated with Paget's disease of bone: a population-based study. J Bone Miner Res 2008;23(6):819–25.
[9] Singer FR. Paget disease: when to treat and when not to treat. Nat Rev Rheumatol 2009;5(9):483–9.
[10] Meunier PJ, Vignon E. Therapeutic strategy in Paget's disease of bone. Bone 1999;17(Suppl. 5):489S–491SS.

[11] Selby PL, Davie MW, Ralston SH, Stone MD. Guidelines on the management of Paget's disease of bone. Bone 2002;31(3):366–73.
[12] Josse RG, Hanley DA, Kendler D, Ste Marie LG, Adachi JD, Brown J. Diagnosis and treatment of Paget's disease of bone. Clin Invest Med 2007;30(5):E210–23.
[13] Lyles KW, Siris ES, Singer FR, Meunier PJ. A clinical approach to diagnosis and management of Paget's disease of bone. J Bone Miner Res 2001;16(8):1379–87.
[14] Brown JP, Chines AA, Myers WR, Eusebio RA, Ritter-Hrncirik C, Hayes CW. Improvement of pagetic bone lesions with risedronate treatment: a radiologic study. Bone 2000;26(3):263–7.
[15] Brown JP, Hosking DJ, Ste-Marie L, et al. Risedronate, a highly effective, short-term oral treatment for Paget's disease: a dose-response study. Calcif Tissue Int 1999;64(2):93–9.
[16] Brown JP. Metabolic bone diseases: treating Paget disease: when matters more than how. Nat Rev Rheumatol 2009;5(12):663–5.
[17] Langston AL, Campbell MK, Fraser WD, et al. Randomized trial of intensive bisphosphonate treatment versus symptomatic management in Paget's disease of bone. J Bone Miner Res 2010;25(1):20–31.
[18] Reid IR, Cundy T, Bolland MJ, Grey A. Response to publication of PRISM trial. J Bone Miner Res 2010;25(6):1463–4 author reply 5–6.
[19] Vasireddy S, Talwalkar A, Miller H, Mehan R, Swinson DR. Patterns of pain in Paget's disease of bone and their outcomes on treatment with pamidronate. Clin Rheumatol 2003;22(6):376–80.
[20] Hadjipavlou AG, Gaitanis IN, Kontakis GM. Paget's disease of the bone and its management. J Bone Joint Surg Br 2002;84(2):160–9.
[21] Tan A, Ralston SH. Clinical presentation of Paget's disease: evaluation of a contemporary cohort and systematic review. Calcif Tissue Int 2014;95(5):385–92.
[22] Parvizi J, Frankle MA, Tiegs RD, Sim FH. Corrective osteotomy for deformity in Paget disease. J Bone Joint Surg Am 2003;85-A(4):697–702.
[23] Theodorou DJ, Theodorou SJ, Kakitsubata Y. Imaging of Paget disease of bone and its musculoskeletal complications: self-assessment module. AJR Am J Roentgenol 2011;196(Suppl. 6):WS53–6.
[24] Melton 3rd LJ, Tiegs RD, Atkinson EJ, O'Fallon WM. Fracture risk among patients with Paget's disease: a population-based cohort study. J Bone Miner Res 2000;15 (11):2123–8.
[25] Rasmussen JM, Hopfensperger ML. Placement and restoration of dental implants in a patient with Paget's disease in remission: literature review and clinical report. J Prosthodont: Official J Am College Prosthodont 2008;17(1):35–40.
[26] Wegrzyn J, Pibarot V, Chapurlat R, Carret JP, Bejui-Hugues J, Guyen O. Cementless total hip arthroplasty in Paget's disease of bone: a retrospective review. Int Orthop 2010;34(8):1103–9.
[27] Mangham DC, Davie MW, Grimer RJ. Sarcoma arising in Paget's disease of bone: declining incidence and increasing age at presentation. Bone 2009;44(3):431–6.
[28] Deyrup AT, Montag AG, Inwards CY, Xu Z, Swee RG, Krishnan Unni K. Sarcomas arising in Paget disease of bone: a clinicopathologic analysis of 70 cases. Arch Pathol Lab Med 2007;131(6):942–6.
[29] Lopez C, Thomas DV, Davies AM. Neoplastic transformation and tumour-like lesions in Paget's disease of bone: a pictorial review. Eur Radiol 2003;13(Suppl. 4): L151–63.
[30] Poncelet A. The neurologic complications of Paget's disease. J Bone Miner Res 1999;14(Suppl. 2):88–91.
[31] Dabbs TR, Skjodt K. Prevalence of angioid streaks and other ocular complications of Paget's disease of bone. Br J Ophthalmol 1990;74(10):579–82.

[32] Monsell EM. The mechanism of hearing loss in Paget's disease of bone. Laryngoscope 2004;114(4):598–606.
[33] Saifuddin A, Hassan A. Paget's disease of the spine: unusual features and complications. Clin Radiol 2003;58(2):102–11.
[34] Hultgren HN. Osteitis deformans (Paget's disease) and calcific disease of the heart valves. Am J Cardiol 1998;81(12):1461–4.
[35] Laroche M, Delmotte A. Increased arterial calcification in Paget's disease of bone. Calcif Tissue Int 2005;77(3):129–33.
[36] Brandi ML, Falchetti A. What is the relationship between Paget's disease of bone and hyperparathyroidism? J Bone Miner Res 2006;21(Suppl. 2):P69–74.
[37] Lyles KW, Gold DT, Newton RA, et al. Peyronie's disease is associated with Paget's disease of bone. J Bone Miner Res 1997;12(6):929–34.
[38] Merlotti D, Gennari L, Galli B, et al. Characteristics and familial aggregation of Paget's disease of bone in Italy. J Bone Miner Res 2005;20(8):1356–64.

CHAPTER 9

Treatment of Paget's Disease of Bone

Ian R. Reid[1,2]
[1]Faculty of Medical and Health Sciences, University of Auckland, Auckland, New Zealand
[2]Auckland District Health Board, Auckland, New Zealand

INTRODUCTION

Paget's disease is a chronic, uni- or multifocal condition of increased bone turnover, involving overactivity of both osteoblasts and osteoclasts. These changes in cellular activity can result in local bone loss or in the deposition of increased amounts of low quality "woven" bone. It is not clear whether the causative lesion involves primarily 'blasts or 'clasts, but therapies have generally been antiosteoclastic (antiresorptive) because these are the only pharmaceuticals that have been available. There is tight coupling between 'blasts and 'clasts, so antiresorptive therapies lead to rapid decreases in osteoclast activity followed, after a period of 2−3 months, by similar declines in osteoblast activity. The treatment of Paget's disease is now virtually always with a potent bisphosphonate, typically zoledronate since this has the highest rates of biochemical response and the greatest longevity of these responses. The most commonly used test for monitoring disease activity is serum alkaline phosphatase, which is a measure of osteoblast activity. Because of the tight coupling of 'blasts and 'clasts, measures of either type of cellular activity are quite acceptable, as long as the time lag in response is kept in mind.

ANTIPAGETIC MEDICATIONS

Calcitonin

The first antiosteoclast treatment to be widely used in Paget's disease was calcitonin, a peptide hormone secreted by the C-cells in the thyroid, which binds directly to its receptor on the osteoclast surface and inhibits osteoclast activity. With repeated injections, numbers of osteoclasts are decreased. While a number of calcitonins have been used in the past, salmon calcitonin is the only available preparation in most countries at

S.V. Reddy (Ed): Advances in Pathobiology and Management of Paget's Disease of Bone.
DOI: http://dx.doi.org/10.1016/B978-0-12-805083-5.00009-9

present, and is typically administered as a daily subcutaneous injection of 100 IU. Parenteral calcitonin reduces biochemical markers of bone turnover by 40–50% and produces radiological improvement [1]. While this was a signal advance when it first became available, complete control of disease activity is seldom achieved and relapse occurs rapidly following treatment cessation. In some patients resistance to the effects of calcitonin develops despite continued administration of the drug, probably as a result of the development of antibodies to calcitonin [2]. The use of daily injections and the frequent occurrence of side-effects (such as nausea and flushing) limit its acceptability to patients [3]. As a result of its limited efficacy and lower acceptability to patients, calcitonin has been supplanted by the bisphosphonates, except in the rare instances when these are contraindicated.

Bisphosphonates

The bisphosphonates are a class of antiresorptive drugs with a high affinity for bone, which are preferentially taken up at sites of high turnover. As a result, they are concentrated into pagetic lesions. The bisphosphonate nucleus consists of two phosphate groups joined through a central carbon atom. This P–C–P bond is very stable and is not subject to metabolism in humans. The cluster of oxygen atoms associated with the bisphosphonate nucleus confers a strong negative charge which results in avid binding of the bisphosphonate to the positively charged surface of bone. During bone resorption the bisphosphonate is ingested by osteoclasts. Once inside the cell, most bisphosphonates inhibit the enzyme, farnesyl pyrophosphate synthase, a critical step in the mevalonate pathway which leads to the synthesis of cholesterol. Disruption of this pathway adversely affects the osteoclast cytoskeleton, thus inhibiting bone resorption and, when present in high concentrations, resulting in osteoclast apoptosis. For most bisphosphonates, clinical potency is determined by both their affinity for hydroxyapatite (which determines skeletal uptake) and the potency of their inhibition of this target enzyme [4,5]. In contrast, etidronate interferes with the formation of ATP, thus impairing osteoclast activity. In vitro affinity for hydroxyapatite also impacts on the longevity of the antiosteoclastic effect, with avidly bound agents producing more sustained inhibition of bone resorption in clinical studies [5].

Etidronate was the first bisphosphonate to be used in Paget's disease and it produced larger and longer lasting effects on bone turnover than the calcitonins [6,7]. Various dosing regimens were found to be comparably effective, and efficacy was mainly determined by the total dose [8,9]. However, the high doses necessary to control disease activity in some patients, resulted in the development of osteomalacia. This caused bone pain and low trauma fractures, though it resolved following drug withdrawal [7,10,11]. Osteomalacia appeared to result from a pyrophosphate-like effect of etidronate inhibiting hydroxyapatite crystal formation. To overcome this problem, other bisphosphonates were developed which dissociated the antiosteoclastic and mineralization inhibiting properties of these drugs.

Clodronate [12] and *tiludronate* [13] achieved this to some extent, but these were quickly eclipsed by the much more potent amino-bisphosphonates, which contained a nitrogen atom in the side-chain. The Leiden group pioneered this development, and demonstrated normalization of bone resorption within 1 week with oral *pamidronate*, though normalization of bone formation lagged behind by 3–6 months [14]. These changes in cell activity were confirmed on bone biopsy, and healing of lytic radiologic lesions was subsequently demonstrated [15] (Fig. 9.1). Oral pamidronate produced an unacceptable frequency of upper gastrointestinal symptoms, so it has mainly been used intravenously, a short course of infusions producing biochemical remissions lasting 2–3 years [16]. Pamidronate has now been outmoded by more potent amino-bisphosphonates.

Alendronate has one more carbon atom in its side chain than pamidronate, and this substantially increases its antiresorptive potency. It was primarily developed for treatment of osteoporosis, but was also assessed in two Paget's disease randomized trials, one comparing it to placebo [17] and the other to etidronate [18]. Alendronate 40 mg/day for 6 months normalized alkaline phosphatase in 60–70% of subjects, led to healing of lytic radiologic lesions, and restored normal lamellar bone histology in the place of woven bone (Fig. 9.2). These were critical demonstrations of the ability of bisphosphonates to arrest disease progression rather than just modify biochemical markers. There was no evidence of impaired bone mineralization, in contrast to etidronate. Follow-up of these patients has demonstrated the longevity of responses to alendronate, all the more so when the drug was administered for 12 months rather than 6 [19]. Therefore, alendronate has been widely used in Paget's disease over the last decade, the 6-month courses being repeated as necessary, typically at intervals of 2–5 years.

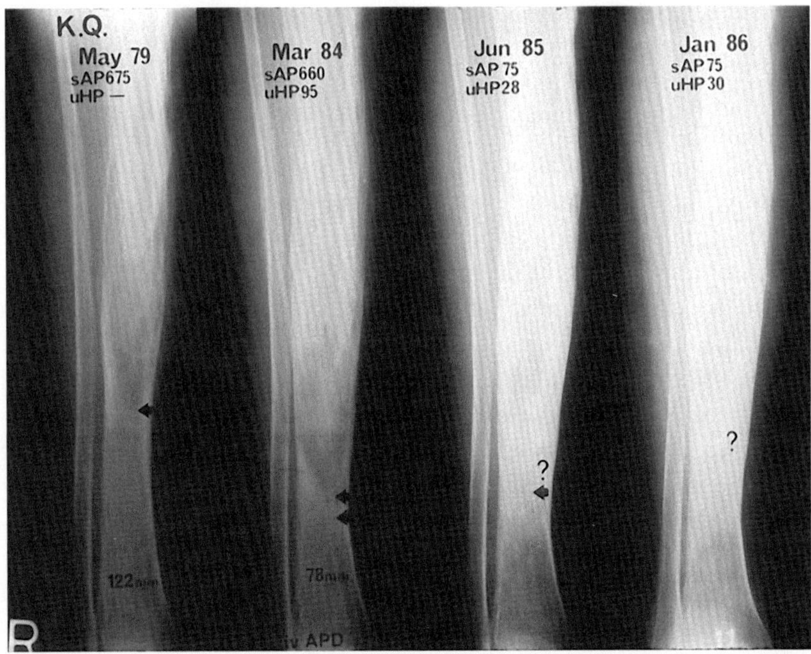

Figure 9.1 Sequence of radiographs demonstrating the progression of a lytic lesion in the tibia of an untreated patient between May 1979 and Mar. 1984. A course of intravenous pamidronate was administered in Mar. 1984, and radiographs over the following 2 years demonstrated complete healing of the lytic lesion with no suggestion of relapse, even though the patient had no further therapy. *Radiographs supplied by Prof. HK Ibbertson. Copyright IR Reid, used with permission.*

Risedronate (30 mg/day for 2–3 months) was evaluated in open studies [20–22] and in a randomized trial comparing it with etidronate [23]. The decision to use it for shorter treatment periods than alendronate is arbitrary, and the optimal course length has not been rigorously determined for either agent. Alkaline phosphatase was normalized in 73% of patients, and risedronate was shown to relieve pagetic pain (though the effects were not significant between-groups). Upper gastrointestinal side-effects continued to be an issue, but less so than with pamidronate, possibly because the doses administered were much smaller. However, this problem motivated further development of intravenous bisphosphonates.

Ibandronate has been shown to be very effective in short-term control of Paget's disease activity [24] but has not been actively marketed for this indication. Recent work has focused on single-dose therapy with intravenous *zoledronate* (also referred to as zoledronic acid), the most potent

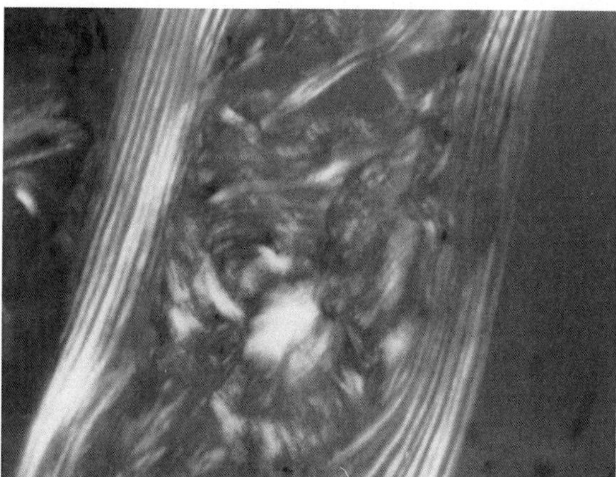

Figure 9.2 Section of a bone trabecula affected by Paget's disease, viewed under polarized light to show orientation of lamellae. In the center of the trabecula the collagen fibers are chaotically laid down (woven bone) consistent with active Paget's disease. Over the outer surfaces, collagen is organized in parallel lamellae, indicating the restoration of normal bone microarchitecture following treatment with alendronate. *Reprinted with permission from: Reid IR, et al. Biochemical and radiologic improvement in Paget's disease of bone treated with alendronate—a randomized, placebo-controlled trial. Am J Med 1996;101:341–8.*

bisphosphonate in clinical use. This high clinical potency results from potent inhibition of farnesyl pyrophosphate synthase and high affinity for hydroxyapatite [4,5]. A single intravenous dose of zoledronate 5 mg was compared with a two-month course of oral risedronate 30 mg/day in two clinical trials, combined into a single study report [25]. In the 6-month core study, 96% of patients randomized to zoledronate showed a therapeutic response (based on serum alkaline phosphatase changes) compared with 74% of those randomized to risedronate ($p < 0.001$). Alkaline phosphatase levels normalized in 89% of patients in the zoledronate group and 58% of those given risedronate ($p < 0.001$). Zoledronate showed a more rapid onset of action, and superior effects on quality of life measures, including pain relief.

The patients who showed a therapeutic response to either intervention in the core study were invited to enter a follow-up study to determine the duration of remission without further intervention. Two years after drug administration, therapeutic response was maintained in 98% of those receiving zoledronate but in only 57% of risedronate-treated patients [26], and at 6 years these figures were 87% and 38%, respectively [27]. Bone turnover data from this study are shown in Fig. 9.3, and show a dramatic fall after the single infusion of zoledronate with the mean value remaining

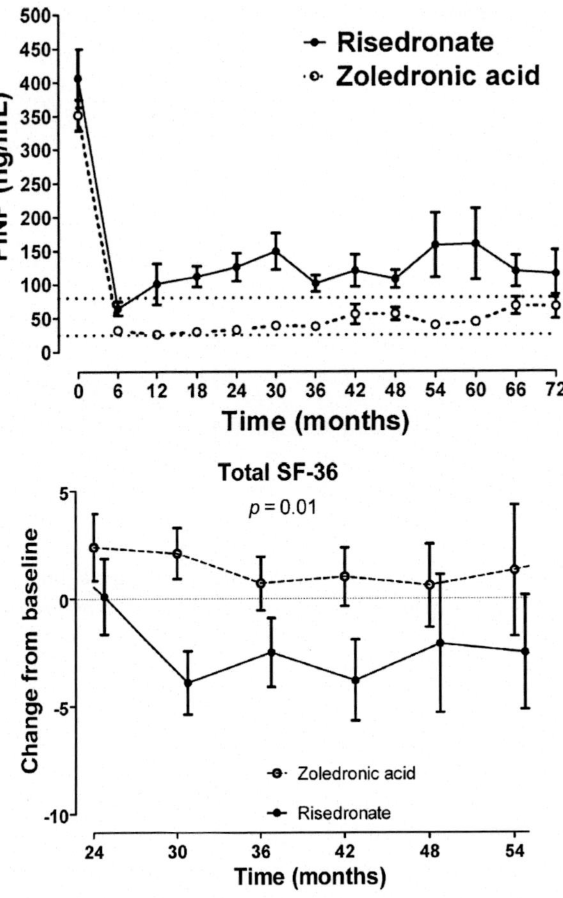

Figure 9.3 Upper panel: Serum PINP in patients with Paget's disease treated with either a single infusion of zoledronate or a 2-month course of risedronate 30 mg/day, at baseline. Data are mean ± SEM. Reference ranges are shown as broken horizontal lines. PINP was significantly lower in the zoledronate group compared with risedronate from 12 to 66 months inclusive. It should be noted that once an individual met the criterion for relapse or received further therapy for Paget's disease, the protocol stipulated that they were withdrawn from the study. Therefore, turnover markers in the risedronate group do not progressively rise, since there is a steady attrition of relapsing patients from that group.
Lower panel: Changes in total SF-36 scores from baseline (mean ± SE). A negative change indicates worse quality of life. The between-groups comparison is based on analysis of covariance ($p = 0.01$). *Reprinted from Reid et al. J Bone Miner Res 2011, used with permission.*

within the normal range throughout the follow-up period. The gradual upward trend in turnover in the zoledronate group arose substantially from increases in patients in the top quartile, while the majority of subjects showed stable values to the end of follow-up. Disease activity at 6 months was predictive of subsequent outcome—patients with serum alkaline phosphatase <80 U/L or procollagen type I N-terminal propeptide (PINP) <40 μg/L at this time have a 7–8% risk of relapse in the following 6.5 years. Paralleling this superior biochemical control, was a sustained improvement in quality of life scores in the zoledronate patients compared with those having had risedronate (Fig. 9.3, lower panel) [27].

These data pose the question as to whether this response is just a very sustained suppressive effect, or whether some patients might have actually been "cured." We have carried out bone scintigrams in a few patients remaining in biochemical remission at >5 years after a single infusion of zoledronate to gain insight into this question. In some, lesions have not reactivated whereas in others there are very low levels of activity seen, suggesting that disease reactivation will eventually become apparent. The series of scintigrams in Fig. 9.4, span a period of 7 years after a zoledronate infusion. There is a suggestion of persistence of minor activity in the

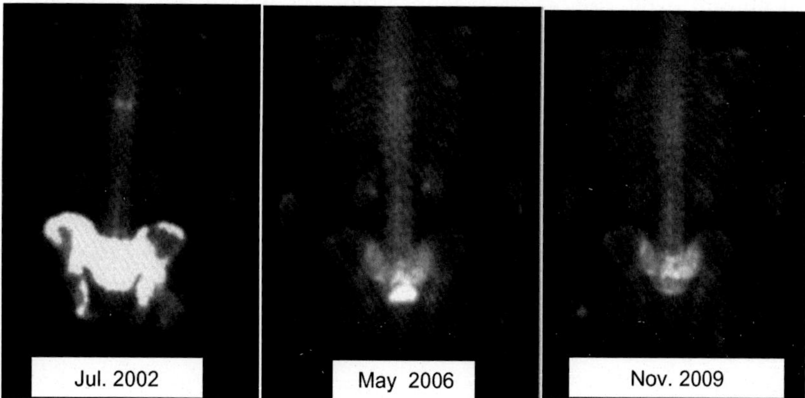

Figure 9.4 Sequence of bone scintigrams in a patient with Paget's disease, immediately before treatment with zoledronate 5 mg (Jul. 2002), and then at 4 and 7 years afterwards, without further intervention. At baseline, intense activity is seen throughout most of the pelvis, and a small focus of disease in a mid-thoracic vertebra. There is slight reactivation in the sacrum in 2009, but not in the thoracic spine. *Reprinted from Reid et al. J Bone Miner Res 2011, used with permission.*

Table 9.1 Standard regimens for drugs used in the treatment of Paget's disease

Drug	Usual regimen
Zoledronate	One intravenous infusion of 5 mg over 15 min
Risedronate	30 mg/day for 2 months
Alendronate	40 mg/day for 6 months
Pamidronate	30 mg/day intravenously over 4 h for 3 days
Clodronate	400–1600 mg/day orally for 3–6 months or 300 mg/day intravenously for 5 days
Tiludronate	400 mg/day for 3 months
Etidronate	400 mg/day for 3 months
Salmon calcitonin	100 U sc or im daily

sacrum at 3.5 and 7 years, but there is no sign of reactivation of the lesion in the thoracic spine, suggesting that in the same patient some lesions might be cured while others are only markedly suppressed.

The exact mechanism for this sustained efficacy remains uncertain, but it may be contributed to by the delivery of the entire drug dose in one bolus at a time when lesional uptake of bisphosphonate is maximal. In contrast, when dosing is spread over months there is a progressive diminution in bone turnover, accompanied by a parallel reduction in bisphosphonate uptake into the pagetic lesion. A single-dose strategy might both eliminate the cohort of pagetic osteoclasts within the pagetic focus but also destroy other cells within the lesion, including any putative osteoblast or stem cell clone which is driving the increased osteoclastogenesis. We have recently demonstrated that bisphosphonate bound to a bone surface is toxic not only to osteoclasts, but to many other cells on that surface [28]. The high potency and bone affinity of zoledronate maximize both the acute cytotoxicity and its persistence.

The standard regimens for these antipagetic drugs are set out in Table 9.1.

Safety of Bisphosphonates

Potent bisphosphonates, whether administered orally or intravenously, have a good safety profile. When given by mouth, the main issue is upper gastrointestinal irritation, and when given intravenously a flu-like illness occurs in about 25% of subjects [25]. It is important to note that the manifestations of this response are more diverse than has previously been recognized [29], and that uveitis and other forms of eye inflammation are probably a part of this. Bisphosphonate-associated uveitis is promptly responsive to topical steroids [30], and is not necessarily a contraindication to retreatment, particularly since all aspects of the flu-like illness are much less common on redosing [29]. Intravenous bisphosphonates are potentially nephrotoxic, so assessing renal function before dosing is important, and zoledronate should not be administered if the glomerular filtration rate is <30 mL/minute. Potent bisphosphonates can produce symptomatic hypocalcemia in individuals with marked vitamin D deficiency (25-hydroxyvitamin D <25 nmol/L). In patients at risk of vitamin D deficiency, supplementation prior to treatment is advisable, if necessary with a single large oral dose (eg, calciferol 100,000 units) [31,32].

The much rarer but more serious side-effects of bisphosphonates do not appear to be a significant issue in the treatment of Paget's disease. There have been isolated case reports of osteonecrosis of the jaw [33] and a subtrochanteric fracture [34] which may well have been related to pagetic deformity rather than bisphosphonate. In the two largest clinical trials of bisphosphonates in this condition, no cases of either problem were reported [25,35] even with follow-up beyond 6 years [27].

With all bisphosphonates other than zoledronate, the doses required to achieve disease control in Paget's disease have been higher than those required for the management of osteoporosis. With the discovery that only a single dose of zoledronate is necessary for sustained disease control in Paget's disease (in comparison with the annual dosing required in osteoporosis) the implication is that long-term safety concerns are even less in Paget's disease. This is particularly reassuring, since it has now been demonstrated that zoledronate has a good safety profile even after nine annual doses [36].

Future Medicines

New antiresorptive drugs continue to be developed for the treatment of osteoporosis and of cancers metastatic to bone. These agents have potential utility in the management of Paget's disease, though there is very little published experience available. Denosumab is a monoclonal antibody directed against RANK-ligand. If Paget's disease is truly a clonal expansion of osteoclast-like cells, then denosumab would not be expected to be an effective drug, since it is directed at the development of osteoclasts from preosteoclasts. However, one published case report [37] and unpublished anecdotes suggest that denosumab does substantially reduce bone turnover in Paget's disease. How durable these improvements are is unknown—the antibody only persists in the circulation for about 6 months after the subcutaneous injection, so it may not achieve the prolonged remissions that are possible with bisphosphonates. The use of cathepsin K inhibitors in Paget's disease has not yet been described. Their rapid offset of action suggests that continuous therapy would be necessary if they did prove to be effective in this area.

WHOM TO TREAT

Since the advent of the first effective treatments for Paget's disease, clinicians have been faced with the question of whom they should treat and what the treatment endpoints should be. The answers to these questions have evolved over the last 40 years and are influenced by treatment efficacy, cost, side-effects, and the likelihood that treatment will modify the long-term disease course. While the calcitonins and the bisphosphonates impact on bone turnover markers, there is not necessarily merit in reducing bone turnover if this does not translate into some symptomatic benefit for the patient.

Where the use of an antipagetic therapy results in immediate symptomatic improvement, the decision to treat is straightforward. While many available therapies have not been proven in clinical trials to reduce pagetic pain, it is a common experience that patients with pain localized to a region affected by Paget's disease will experience partial or complete relief of that pain following treatment with calcitonin or a bisphosphonate. This is particularly true of bone pain, but there is also frequently improvement in pain from joints with adjacent pagetic changes, and any residual pain in this context is usually attributed to secondary osteoarthritis. With calcitonin, biochemical and symptomatic improvements did not extend much beyond the duration of therapy, so the balance of symptomatic improvement against side-effects and costs have only to be judged over the short term.

With the advent of the bisphosphonates, and the demonstration of significant biochemical improvement extending well beyond the period of intervention, came the question of whether more intensive therapy was appropriate to modify long-term disease progression and prevent complications. The limited number of clinical trials (and their small size and short duration, in most cases) means that a definitive answer to this question is not possible. Only one study has set out to specifically address this question the PRISM trial carried out in the United Kingdom [35]. This study recruited 1324 patients with Paget's disease and randomized them to either "symptomatic" or "intensive" management. In the former, patients were given low potency bisphosphonates or calcitonin for symptomatic disease, though this could be escalated to potent bisphosphonates if necessary. The comparator group was intensive therapy, in which patients were treated with potent bisphosphonates, usually risedronate, with a view to normalization of serum alkaline phosphatase. Seventy percent of patients entering the study had already received bisphosphonate treatment, and as a result, disease activity at recruitment was not particularly high (mean alkaline phosphatase ~135% of the upper limit of normal (ULN)). At the end of the study, after a mean duration of follow-up of 3 years, mean alkaline phosphatase in the intensive therapy group was 80% ULN, and that in the symptomatic group was 110% ULN. Thus, only a small difference in disease activities was achieved, so it is possibly not surprising that there were no differences in the number of pagetic complications that occurred in this study. It should be noted that, while the general aim of the PRISM study was to determine whether disease complications could be prevented, in fact the study was powered to assess the reduction in total numbers of fractures (not just fractures through pagetic bone), which was a curious endpoint to choose since fracture is mainly a complication of osteoporosis, a condition that the trial participants were not suffering from. Intensive therapy, however, did diminish the need for analgesics. The shortcomings and inconsistencies of the PRISM trial need to be borne in mind when its negative results are used as evidence of the futility of aiming for remission of disease activity in Paget's disease.

A second approach to assessing the value of disease suppression and preventing complications is to consider what we know of the natural history of the condition, and the evidence available that treatment interferes with the components of this natural history. There is extensive, though anecdotal, documentation of the progression of pagetic lesions, particularly in long bones. This has been systematically quantified to progress at about 1 cm/year [38]. Radiographic records show (eg, Fig. 9.5) that this progression is led by a lytic front which, over time, transforms into sclerotic and deformed bone which remains as a permanent residuum. The radiographic appearance of lysis results from large numbers of osteoclasts increasing bone resorption, sclerosis results from osteoblast overabundance, and the deformity is contributed to by dysregulation of cell activity and the resulting deposition of mechanically inferior woven bone. Therapy has been shown to address each of these pathogenic components. Potent bisphosphonates dramatically reduce bone resorption, assessed biochemically and on bone biopsies [17], which results in the healing of

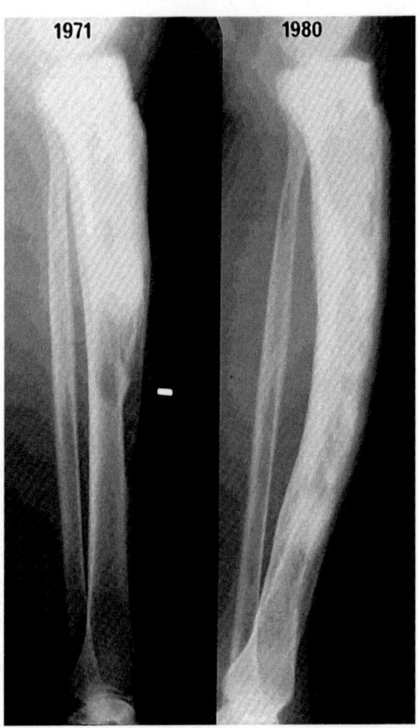

Figure 9.5 Tibia affected by Paget's disease. The upper tibia is of increased density and width as a result of osteoblast overactivity, whereas the lower part of the affected bone shows a lytic region resulting from osteoclastic bone resorption. Below this, the bone is normal. Between 1971 and 1980 there was progression of the disease down the tibia, with a bowing deformity resulting from this. *Radiographs supplied by Prof. HK Ibbertson. Copyright IR Reid, used with permission.*

radiographic lytic lesions (Fig. 9.1). This has been demonstrated both in case series [15] and in a randomized, controlled trial [17]. Histologically, the reduced bone turnover associated with therapy results in the laying down of normal lamellar bone in place of the mechanically inferior woven bone produced when the disease is active [17] (Fig. 9.2). Thus, the well-documented progression of radiographic changes along a bone is halted. As demonstrated in Fig. 9.5, radiographic disease progression is associated with the development of deformity so it is reasonable to infer that halting disease progression will limit the development of new deformity, with its possible consequences of osteoarthritis and fracture. While trials are not available which have adequately addressed fracture numbers or the need for joint replacement, the demonstrated efficacy in restoring normal histology and preventing radiological progression, make it reasonable to infer that these late sequelae are also likely to be reduced. It is likely that the long-term improvement in quality of life found in the zoledronate phase 3 trial programme is contributed to by this arrest of disease progression, as well as by the acute decreases in pain that were observed in the first 6 months of the study.

As a result of these considerations, a number of experts and consensus groups have recommended that not only should symptomatic Paget's disease be treated, but also treatment should be provided when the site of the pagetic process and the patient's life expectancy together provide a reasonable likelihood that disease complications will ensue [3,39,40]. Thus, treatment is recommended for active lesions in long bones particularly those that are weight-bearing (which are likely to bow and/or fracture), juxta-articular Paget's disease (likely to result in premature osteoarthritis), vertebral disease (which may impinge on nerve roots and/or rarely cause paraplegia), and skull Paget's disease (which can result in headaches, deformity and, with involvement of the temporal bone, deafness). If a patient is asymptomatic and has Paget's disease at a site which poses a very low risk of complications, then simple observation may be a reasonable strategy.

The sustained normalization of biochemical and scintigraphic indices of disease activity produced by zoledronate has resulted in much less frequent follow-up being necessary in patients following treatment with this drug, and this introduces a more pragmatic argument in favor of intervention. In patients with active disease, it may be cheaper to treat and thus reduce the frequency of follow-up assessments than to leave the patient untreated, and closely monitor disease progression. The cost-effectiveness of this approach is dependent on the cost of zoledronate and its infusion, which vary between countries. However, the availability of generic zoledronate is likely to result in substantial decreases in drug costs, making this approach increasingly attractive. The fact that the use of zoledronate in patients with biochemical evidence of disease activity has been shown to result in sustained improvements in quality of life is a further important reason for favoring a more interventionist approach [27].

MONITORING

The appropriate follow-up of a patient with Paget's disease is dependent on the skeletal sites affected and the degree of disease activity. For instance, in an asymptomatic patient with minimal abnormality of bone turnover markers, who has disease in the pelvis, but well away from the hip joints, in whom clinical, radiological, and biochemical status has been stable for a number of years, review at intervals of several years with a clinical examination and check of serum alkaline phosphatase may be all that is needed. At the other extreme, is the individual with incipient paraplegia, in whom vigorous intervention, follow-up biochemistry over succeeding weeks, and even regular monitoring of bone scintigraphy to ensure that local disease activity has been eliminated, may be appropriate.

A more common scenario would be the patient who has been treated with their first course of bisphosphonate. In this situation, I would usually see them 6 months after treatment and monitor their clinical response (resolution of pagetic pain, side-effects from medication), relevant examination findings (eg, local tenderness, warmth over an affected tibia, range of movement at an affected joint), and biochemistry (typically I measure serum total alkaline phosphatase and serum PINP, since the latter is slightly more sensitive to detecting changes in disease activity than the former [24]). If biochemistry has been reduced to the lower half of the normal range by treatment, the patient has no ongoing symptoms, and is considered at low immediate risk of complications, then I would probably review them again in about 2–4 years' time.

In the patient who remains in clinical and biochemical remission 5–6 years after a first dose of zoledronate, I often repeat bone scintigraphy, since this allows a more precise estimate of disease activity. If the lesion is inactive scintigraphically 5 years after treatment, then it is highly likely that it will not become clinically relevant in the subsequent 5 years, and follow-up can be scheduled accordingly.

There are some situations that require much closer follow-up. One such, is the presence of a lytic lesion, particularly if it is in a weight-bearing bone, where there is a significant risk of fracture. If this is the only skeletal site affected, biochemical markers may be normal and not indicative of disease activity. It is sensible to follow these lesions with plain radiographs till healing is confirmed, and again scintigraphy may be very helpful in guiding the need for further intervention.

The advent of single dose zoledronate treatment has profoundly changed the frequency and intensity of follow-up. Following oral courses of potent agents such as risedronate and alendronate, it is common to review patients at intervals of 6–12 months, and expect to retreat at intervals of 2–4 years.

ANALGESICS

Paget's disease can cause bone and joint pain, so general measures to address this, including analgesics, are appropriate. However, pain relief only lasts as long as the analgesic drugs are taken, whereas potent bisphosphonates can provide sustained relief of pain without further dosing. Also, analgesics do not address the underlying disease process, so joint damage or bone deformity are likely to progress. For these reasons, analgesics should be regarded as adjunctive therapies only. In practice, they are rarely required for pagetic bone pain since this is rapidly responsive to bisphosphonates.

SURGERY

Disease complications sometimes require surgical intervention. Joint replacement, particularly of the hip or knee, is common, since juxta-articular deformity results in premature arthritis. Osteotomy may be required to correct long bone deformity, and fractures may require surgical management. The indications for these interventions are similar to those in a nonpagetic population. Rarely, Paget's disease of a vertebral body will be associated with paraplegia. Spinal cord compression may contribute to this problem, but diversion of the local blood supply away from the spinal cord to the pagetic vertebra may be a key contributor to the development of a neurological deficit [41]. Surgical management of this problem has been associated with very poor outcomes, whereas intensive bisphosphonate therapy will often result in substantial neurological improvement [42].

Pagetic bone is very vascular, reflecting the high metabolic activity of the affected bone cells. As a result, it bleeds profusely during surgery and hemostasis can be difficult. Therefore, patients with active disease should be treated before undergoing surgery on affected bone in order to reduce blood loss. While this has not been subjected to clinical trials it is endorsed by expert opinion [3,39].

A caution to keep in mind when undertaking orthopedic surgery on pagetic patients is that Paget's disease can be transplanted with a bone graft [43]. The iliac crest is a common donor site for grafts and also a common site for Paget's disease.

Disclosure

Ian Reid has received research funding and consulting fees from Novartis, Merck, and Amgen.

Supported by the Health Research Council of New Zealand.

REFERENCES

[1] Doyle FH, Greenberg PB, Joplin GF, MacIntyre I. Radiological evidence of a dose-related response to long-term treatment of Paget's disease with human calcitonin. Br J Radiol 1974;47:1–8.

[2] Singer FR, Aldred JP, Neer RM, Krane SM, John T, Potts J, et al. An evaluation of antibodies and clinical resistance to salmon calcitonin. J Clin Invest 1972;51:2331–8.

[3] Delmas PD, Meunier PJ. The management of Paget's disease of bone. N Engl J Med 1997;336(8):558–66.

[4] Dunford JE, Thompson K, Coxon FP, et al. Structure-activity relationships for inhibition of farnesyl diphosphate synthase in vitro and inhibition of bone resorption in vivo by nitrogen-containing bisphosphonates. J Pharmacol Exp Ther 2001;296 (2):235–42.

[5] Nancollas GH, Tang R, Phipps RJ, et al. Novel insights into actions of bisphosphonates on bone: differences in interactions with hydroxyapatite. Bone 2006;38 (5):617–27.

[6] Altman RD, Johnston CC, Khairi MR, Wellman H, Serafini AN, Sankey RR. Influence of disodium etidronate on clinical and laboratory manifestations of Paget's disease of bone (osteitis deformans). N Engl J Med 1973;289(26):1379–84.

[7] Smith R, Russell RGG, Bishop MC, Woods CG, Bishop M. Paget's disease of bone: experience with a diphosphonate (disodium etidronate) in treatment. Q J Med 1973;42:235–56.

[8] de Vries HR, Bijvoet OLM. Results of prolonged treatment of Paget's disease of bone with disodiun ethane-1-hydroxy-1, 1-diphosphonate (EHDP). Neth J Med 1974;17:281–98.

[9] Khairi MRA, Johnston CC, Altman RD, Wellman HN, Serafini AN, Sankey RR. Treatment of Paget's disease of bone (osteitis deformans). JAMA 1974;28:562–7.

[10] Kantrowitz FG, Byrne MH, Schiller AL, Krane SM. Clinical and biochemical effects of diphosphonates in Paget's diseasde of bone. Arthritis Rheum 1975;18:407.

[11] Khairi MRA, Altman RD, De Rosa GP, Zimmermann J, Schenk RK, Johnston CC. Sodium etidronate in the treatment of Paget's disease of bone: a study of long term results. Ann Intern Med 1977;87:656–63.

[12] Yates AJP, Gray RES, Urwin GH, et al. Intravenous clodronate in the treatment and retreatment of Paget's disease of bone. Lancet 1985;325:1474–7.

[13] Reginster JY, Colson F, Morlock G, Combe B, Ethgen D, Geusens P. Evaluation of the efficacy and safety of oral tiludronate in Paget's disease of bone. A double-blind, multiple-dosage, placebo-controlled study. Arthritis Rheum 1992;35(8):967–74.

[14] Frijlink WB, te Velde J, Bijvoet OLM, Heynen G. Treatment of Paget's disease with (3-amino-1-hydoxypropylidene)-1,1-bisphosphonate (APD). Lancet 1979;i:799–803.

[15] Dodd GW, Ibbertson HK, Fraser TRC, Holdaway IM, Wattie D. Radiological assessment of Paget's disease of bone after treatment with the bisphosphonates EHDP and APD. Br J Radiol 1987;60:849–60.

[16] Harinck HIJ, Papapoulos SE, Blanksma HJ, Moolenaar AJ, Vermeij P, Bijvoet OLM. Paget's disease of bone: early and late responses to three different modes of treatment with aminohydroxypropylidene bisphosphonate (APD). BMJ 1987;295:1301–5.

[17] Reid IR, Nicholson GC, Weinstein RS, et al. Biochemical and radiologic improvement in Paget's disease of bone treated with alendronate—a randomized, placebo-controlled trial. Am J Med 1996;101(4):341–8.

[18] Siris E, Weinstein RS, Altman R, et al. Comparative study of alendronate versus etidronate for the treatment of Paget's disease of bone. J Clin Endocrinol Metab 1996;81(3):961–7.

[19] Cukier KJ, Harrison NJ, Sanders KM, Katowicz MA, Nicholson GC. Long-term remission of Paget's disease after induction of remission with oral alendronate: a fifteen-year follow-up study. International symposium on paget's disease. Oxford: Botnar Institute; 2009.

[20] Hosking DJ, Eusebio RA, Chines AA. Pagets-disease of bone—reduction of disease activity with oral risedronate. Bone 1998;22(1):51–5.

[21] Singer FR, Clemens TL, Eusebio RA, Bekker PJ. Risedronate, a highly effective oral agent in the treatment of patients with severe pagets-disease. J Clin Endocrinol Metab 1998;83(6):1906–10.

[22] Siris ES, Chines AA, Altman RD, et al. Risedronate in the treatment of Pagets-disease of bone—an open label, multicenter study. J Bone Miner Res 1998;13 (6):1032–8.

[23] Miller PD, Brown JP, Siris ES, Hoseyni MS, Axelrod DW, Bekker PJ. A randomized, double-blind comparison of risedronate and etidronate in the treatment of Paget's disease of bone. Am J Med 1999;106(5):513–20.

[24] Reid IR, Davidson JS, Wattie D, et al. Comparative responses of bone turnover markers to bisphosphonate therapy in Paget's disease of bone. Bone 2004;35 (1):224–30.

[25] Reid IR, Miller P, Lyles K, et al. Comparison of a single infusion of zoledronic acid with risedronate for Paget's disease. N Engl J Med 2005;353(9):898–908.

[26] Hosking D, Lyles K, Brown JP, et al. Long-term control of bone turnover in Paget's disease with zoledronic acid and risedronate. J Bone Miner Res 2007;22 (1):142–8.

[27] Reid IR, Lyles K, Su GQ, et al. A single infusion of zoledronic acid produces sustained remissions in Paget disease: data to 6.5 years. J Bone Miner Res 2011;26(9): 2261–70.

[28] Cornish J, Bava U, Callon KE, Bai J, Naot D, Reid IR. Bone-bound bisphosphonate inhibits growth of adjacent non-bone cells. Bone 2011;49:710–16.

[29] Reid IR, Gamble GD, Mesenbrink P, Lakatos P, Black DM. Characterization of and risk factors for the acute-phase response after zoledronic acid. J Clin Endocrinol Metab 2010;95(9):4380–7.

[30] Patel DV, Horne A, House M, Reid IR, McGhee CNJ. The incidence of acute anterior uveitis after intravenous zoledronate. Ophthalmology 2013;120:773–6.

[31] Heaney RP, Armas LAG, Shary JR, Bell NH, Binkley N, Hollis BW. 25-Hydroxylation of vitamin D-3: relation to circulating vitamin D-3 under various input conditions. Am J Clin Nutr 2008;87(6):1738–42.

[32] Lyles KW, Colon-Emeric CS, Magaziner JS, et al. Zoledronic acid and clinical fractures and mortality after hip fracture. N Engl J Med 2007;357(18):1799–809.

[33] Reid IR, Cundy T. Osteonecrosis of the jaw. Skeletal Radiol 2009;38:5–9.

[34] Kilcoyne A, Heffernan EJ. Atypical proximal femoral fractures in patients with Paget disease receiving bisphosphonate therapy. Am J Roentgenol 2011;197(1):W196–7.

[35] Langston AL, Campbell MK, Fraser WD, MacLennan GS, Selby PL, Ralston SH. Randomized trial of intensive bisphosphonate treatment versus symptomatic management in Paget's disease of bone. J Bone Miner Res 2009;25(1):20–31.

[36] Black DM, Reid IR, Cauley JA, et al. The effect of 6 versus 9 years of zoledronic acid treatment in osteoporosis: a randomized second extension to the HORIZON-pivotal fracture trial (PFT). J Bone Miner Res 2015;30(5):934–44.

[37] Schwarz P, Rasmussen AQ, Kvist TM, Andersen UB, Jorgensen NR. Paget's disease of the bone after treatment with Denosumab: a case report. Bone 2012;50(5): 1023–5.

[38] Renier JC, Audran M. Progression in length and width of pagetic lesions, and estimation of age at disease onset. Rev Rhum 1997;64(1):35–43.

[39] Lyles KW, Siris ES, Singer FR, Meunier PJ. A clinical approach to diagnosis and management of Paget's disease of bone. J Bone Miner Res 2001;16(8):1379–87.
[40] Singer FR, Bone III HG, Hosking DJ, et al. Paget's disease of bone: an Endocrine Society Clinical Practice Guideline. J Clin Endocrinol Metab 2014;99(12):4408–22.
[41] McCloskey EV. Neurological complications of Paget's disease. Clin Rev Bone Miner Metab 2002;1:130–43.
[42] Wallace E, Wong JC, Reid IR. Pamidronate treatment of the neurologic sequelae of pagetic spinal stenosis. Arch Int Med 1995;155(16):1813–15.
[43] Hamadouche M, Mathieu M, Topouchian V, De Pinieux G, Courpied JP. Transfer of Paget's disease from one part of the skeleton to another as a result of autogenous bone-grafting—a case report. J Bone Joint Surg 2002;84A(11):2056–61.

INDEX

Note: Page numbers followed by "*f*" and "*t*" refer to figures and tables, respectively.

H

I

J

K

L

M

Q

R

S

T

U

V

W

Z

Printed in the United States
By Bookmasters